INSANITY AND THE INSANE IN POST-FAMINE IRELAND

Mark Finnane

CROOM HELM LONDON

BARNES & NOBLE BOOKS
TOTOWA, NEW JERSEY

© 1981 Mark Finnane
Croom Helm Ltd, 2-10 St John's Road, London SW11

British Library Cataloguing in Publication Data
Finnane, Mark
  Insanity and the insane in post-famine Ireland.
  1. Psychiatric hospitals—Ireland—History
  I. Title
  362.2′1′09415   RC450.173

  ISBN 0-7099-0402-9

First published in the USA 1981 by
BARNES & NOBLE BOOKS
81 ADAMS DRIVE
TOTOWA, New Jersey 07512

Library of Congress Cataloging Card Number: 81-66330

ISBN 0-389-20212-6

To M.K.C.

Printed and bound in Great Britain by
REDWOOD BURN LIMITED
Trowbridge & Esher

83 000698

CONTENTS

TABLES

ABBREVIATIONS

DJMS	*Dublin Journal of Medical Science*
EHR	*Economic History Review*
HC	*House of Commons Papers*
HOS	Hospital records, Public Record Office of Northern Ireland
JMS	*Journal of Mental Science*
MPA	Medico-Psychological Association
MPC	*Medical Press and Circular*
NLI	National Library of Ireland
PRONI	Public Record Office of Northern Ireland
RCPI	Royal College of Physicians in Ireland
RMCB	Male case-book, Richmond Lunatic Asylum
RFCB	Female case-book, Richmond Lunatic Asylum
RP	Chief Secretary's Office, Registered Papers
SPO	State Paper Office, Dublin
SSISI	The journal of the Statistical and Social Inquiry Society of Ireland

Figure 1: District Lunatic Asylums in Ireland, 1870-1898

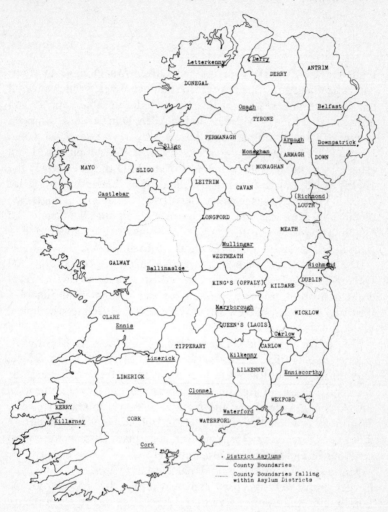

ACKNOWLEDGEMENTS

I am indebted to Barry Smith and Oliver MacDonagh for their encouragement and criticism over the number of years which covered the research and writing of this book. Indispensable support and dialogue have been provided by Judith Allen, Dan Coward, Maureen Finnane, Paul Kauffman and Susan Magarey. Sue Wilson and Patrick Moran advised me about some statistical pitfalls. I am especially grateful to the examiners of the PhD thesis on which the book is based, Ray Brown, Louis Cullen and Kathleen Woodroofe for their comments and suggestions. I have two more long-standing debts: to Beverley Kingston who first agreed with me that the insane and lunatic asylums were subjects worthy of historical analysis; and to Patrick O'Farrell who introduced me to Irish history.

The Research School of Social Sciences at the Australian National University, Canberra, provided excellent conditions and a travel grant for my post-graduate research. My employment in the School of History, University of New South Wales has enabled me to complete the book.

The staff at a number of libraries and record offices have been most helpful. Special thanks are due to those at the State Paper Office, Dublin, the Public Record Office of Northern Ireland, Belfast, the National Library of Ireland, the Library of the Royal College of Physicians in Ireland and the National Library in Canberra. The authorities at a number of hospitals in Ireland helped my inquiries; those at St Brendan's Hospital, Grangegorman, Dublin, were most generous in facilitating my research there.

Maria Giuffre typed the final manuscript with patience and care. Earlier drafts were typed by Janice Aldridge, Karen Gavrilovich, Lois Simms and Bernice Ryan. My thanks are due to all of them.

Mark Finnane

INTRODUCTION

The segregation of the insane in Ireland began quietly. It was not accompanied by dispute between political interests or ideological standpoints. In this it differed significantly from the introduction of the poor law. Neither did such contention appear necessary. At first the asylum was thought likely to affect only a miniscule proportion of the population: a handful of institutions, each of 100 beds or so, would suffice to clear the roads of wandering idiots and the gaols and houses of industry of troublesome lunatics. Once established, however, the asylums continued to expand, seemingly out of the control of central government or local ratepayers. The almost extravagant expansion of asylum accommodation was unique among comparable institutions of social control. As I suggest in this book, the asylum, in both financial and social terms, was rapidly outpacing those monuments of social order, the workhouse and the prison. By the end of the nineteenth century there were empty workhouses in Ireland; the prison population itself had declined sufficiently to allow central government to assume the management of gaols without fear of burdensome financial demands; yet throughout the 1890s and beyond the turn of the century, asylum beds were multiplied, even separate new institutions established. Clearly the asylum possessed great social significance.

Just as the asylum had been introduced to Ireland with relative ease, so it saw, there as elsewhere, no substantial challenge to its existence throughout the century. This legitimacy was ensured by the complicity of Irish society in readily resorting to the use of the state's institutions. To the relatives, friends or neighbours of the committed the asylum offered the possibility of relief from the burden of care, or else from the fear of violence. Moreover, to at least some of the insane the asylum offered refuge from the treacherous and harsh world outside; and it was certainly, I suggest, a more comfortable environment than the nineteenth-century workhouse or prison. To both the state and civil society the asylum became an indispensable part of the social order; their mutual role in bringing this about is a central concern of this study.

Essentially the book covers the period during which the asylum achieved legitimacy and permanency. In the case of Ireland the

search for *origins* is both elusive and instructive. For instance, the establishment of the public asylum there owed much to contemporary developments in England. Rhetoric identical to that abroad in England—of humanitarian concern, of the necessity of classifying the institutionalised poor, criminal and mad, of the superiority of moral therapy to physical remedies—was adopted by the Irish founders. But in the final analysis this rhetoric was of less consequence than the especially powerful position of the state in early nineteenth-century Ireland. What England saw only in 1845, or France in 1838, Ireland had already witnessed in its essentials in 1817: the legislative provision of public asylums for the entire country.[1]

While the English asylum reformers typically held back (or were restrained) from compelling local authorities to provide public asylums, the Irish government showed no such reluctance. I suggest the reasons for this in the first chapter, but the pre-eminent one is worth stating here for its influence lies behind the whole period of this book. The Irish government was, of course, the English government in Ireland. The Catholic majority of Ireland was as yet unrepresented in the Westminster Parliament. In effect Irish affairs were managed by a quasi-colonial administrative structure. The Lord-Lieutenant of Ireland, the Chief Secretary, the Under-Secretary at the Chief Secretary's Office: this triumvirate presided over the fate of Ireland from Dublin Castle, responsible to the Parliament in London rather than to the Irish people. For the most part it was the Chief Secretary who had the upper hand. Between 1812 and 1817 this was the youthful Robert Peel, not a man who was easily persuaded of the necessity of government intervention. Nevertheless, in these years Peel was found ready to assert the power of central government in Ireland. The most notable example consisted of his measures for the policing of Ireland. Another was the move towards the establishment of a system of public asylums. In both cases it was his view, and that of his advisers, that the Irish gentry were incompetent or unwilling to pursue the ameliorative or disciplinary measures necessary to the good government of Ireland.

The significance of this fact—the relative freedom of Dublin Castle to govern in a highly interventionist style in the early nineteenth century—is brought home when we look at the restrictions on government action later in the century. With the achievement of Catholic emancipation and the gradual democratisation of parliamentary representation and local government, Irish affairs could not so readily be dictated from London or the Castle. Indeed it became increasingly

difficult for the authorities in Dublin to carry through initiatives which had already been pursued in Britain. Consequently, while Ireland had taken a leading role in the foundation of asylums it was left in the wake of developments a century later. The laws of committal remained in their mid-nineteenth-century form until 1945 (in the Free State); the physical structures themselves still appeared to a commission of inquiry in the 1960s to bear too glaring a reminder of what was now seen as an inglorious past.[2] As publicly-funded institutions, asylums were particularly vulnerable in the contest between local government and the state as it developed in the later nineteenth and early twentieth centuries. Consequently, while in the early 1900s Britain was stirred by a new discourse on the relation between society and the insane, Ireland remained unmoved: the authority of the state was by this time so seriously compromised that the debate on the 'feeble-minded' passed by without any discernible effect in law or social policy.

Beyond the politics of the asylum this study addresses another set of problems. Uncovering the rudiments of the politics tells us little about the insane themselves. I am concerned, therefore, to establish the social contexts in which nineteenth-century Irish society defined, processed and confined the lunatic. For my purpose these contexts are not biological or psychological problems but those of social history. The law was, of course, essential to the process of confinement, though its role is usually ignored in histories of the asylum. After the Famine the great majority of inmates were committed involuntarily; systematic review of the confined person's status was not a statutory requirement. The whole process of committal was essentially an administrative matter in a judicial framework. It worked, and was for the most part unchallenged, because those in a position of power over the lunatic (the state bureaucracy, the local magistracy or the person's own relative) had every reason to see the process as defensive. Paternalism justified most committals; the safety of the family or neighbourhood justified the rest.

The variety of circumstances in which committal could take place was testimony to the poor definition of the asylum's purpose. This variety continued to expand throughout the nineteenth century. The asylum's population originated in almost every conceivable cause of institutional dependence: forms of physical illness, old age, idiocy, poverty, isolation by the emigration or death of family, excessive drink. The grand categories of madness, mania and melancholia covered a multitude of histories and behaviours. Once inside the walls of the asylum the confined were subjected to classification according

to their degree of intractability, or sent to the infirmary for treatment of physical debility. Perhaps our contemporary distrust of the asylum obviates the necessity for the concluding observations of this book: the tendency to institutional inertia, the transition from paternal care of the ideal asylum to violence exercised against those deemed at law to be not responsible for their actions.

The segregation of the insane, observed the *Journal of Mental Science* in 1856, derived partly from humanity, partly from fear or outraged sensibility.[3] This contained some of the truth. The asylum did not exist because of fear alone, else why bother with anything more than a gaol: humanity, pity, hope for the regeneration of labour lost to society, all contributed to tempering the coercive implications of asylum confinement. All too had their historical context. Fear, certainly, was implicated. At a time when ageing aristocracies and the new bourgeoisie were especially fearful of violence from below, revolutionary or otherwise, 'wandering lunatics' constituted only one object of new instruments of control. In England it was an assault by a lunatic on George III which produced the first 'Dangerous Lunatics' Act. It was a preventive measure, providing for the detention of people who had not committed any crime. The murder of a respectable Dublin merchant in St Stephen's Green 37 years later was the occasion for extending a similar measure to Ireland. From one angle then, the asylum was an unqualified instrument of social control.

But this was not the whole story. The contradictory impulses of this age require also a critical appraisal of the humanitarian motive. In the case of the asylum, the *Journal of Mental Science*'s 'humanity' meant two things. Tory paternalism, most evident in the career of Lord Shaftesbury, the archetype of lunacy reformers, lay on one side: lunacy was essentially providential and the care of the lunatic was one of God's works. A more secular notion of 'humanity' lay behind the endeavour of others. The lunatic's condition was temporary and remediable; his humanity might be recovered through appropriate care such as the provision of a nurturing environment in the shape of the asylum. This was the revolutionary thinking on the lunacy question which informed the parliamentary inquiries from 1815 to 1817. In both its forms the humanitarian persuasion was unable to foresee the malign effects of segregation. The good intentions of the paternalist and the sanguine claims of the moral therapist were stalled by the overcrowding, the routinisation of asylum life, the inevitable impatience, even brutality of staff, in the end by the very mystery of what they were dealing with. Insanity remained an enigma at the end

of the nineteenth century. And in Ireland as much as anywhere else the asylum's history reflected the realities of social power—whether manifested in the priorities and preoccupations of national and local politics, in professionalism, in family life—rather than the attainment of some special knowledge of the constituent elements of sanity and insanity.

Notes

1. On England see Andrew T. Scull, *Museums of Madness: The Social Organization of Insanity in Nineteenth-Century England* (Allen Lane, London, 1979), pp. 107-13; on France, Gerard Bleandonu and Guy Le Gaufey, 'The Creation of the Insane Asylums of Auxerre and Paris' (originally *Annales*, 1975), in R. Forster and O. Ranum (eds.), *Deviants and the Abandoned in French Society* (Johns Hopkins University Press, Baltimore, 1978).

2. Commission of Inquiry on Mental Illness, *Report* (Dublin, 1966), para. 67.

3. *Journal of Mental Science*, vol. 2 (1856), p. 10.

1 ASYLUMS FOR THE LUNATIC POOR, 1817-1867

The early nineteenth century brought a host of institutional innovations to Ireland, brought into Union with Britain in 1800. Confronted with the evidence of social disorder, over-population and an ailing economy, reforming politicians, political economists and social observers, rising professionals, philanthropists and humanitarians of various persuasions and motivations all sought to bring order to Ireland, to foster the conditions in which the transition to a prosperous, capitalist agricultural society might be effected. There were, as Gearóid Ó'Tuathaigh notes, limits to the intervention of the state for the improvement of the condition of the people.[1] The failure of any measure for land reform before the Famine was one such example. Similarly, proposals in the 1830s for state-capitalised employment in the development of the country, or for a state railways system, were soundly defeated by the defenders of the rights of private property.[2]

In other areas, however, the intervention of the state was admissable. So, in the decades following the Union and preceding the Famine, the country's character was transformed by new social institutions. There was a poor law where none had been before, a centrally-directed police force and a reformed magistracy, a system of lunatic asylums considered by many at the time to be the best anywhere. English visitors, though they found much to fault in Ireland, regarded such developments as a reassuring sign of the good being wrought by the government's activity. When he visited Ireland in 1842, William Makepeace Thackeray was much impressed by the Derry lunatic asylum, 'a model of neatness and comfort'. Indeed, he bemoaned the fact that the middle classes could not send their 'afflicted relatives to public institutions of this excellent kind'. The condition of entering

> this admirable asylum is that the patient must be a pauper, and on this account he is supplied with every comfort and the best curative means, and his relations are in perfect security.[3]

Some years later, a colonial administrator spent a few days touring Ireland almost exclusively in visiting police barracks or occasionally calling to view the inmates of the workhouses, still crowded in the aftermath of the Famine.[4] Yet the paradox of a well-developed

18

institutional structure in such a poor economy was also the occasion for remark: Harriet Martineau noted, on her visit to Killarney in 1852, the contrast between the stateliness of the new asylum there (this 'palace' as she described it) and the distressed condition of the peasantry in the countryside nearby.[5] Such a paradox, of course, was inevitable, given the assumptions of Ireland's rulers that only limited areas of social need could be the legitimate object of government intervention.

Nevertheless, in the particular case with which we deal in the following pages, the crucial developments were very much the product of state initiative and control. The ease with which the Irish government after the Union established a comprehensive system of lunatic asylums was facilitated by the 'colonial colour' of that government, as Akenson has argued with respect to the foundation of the Irish education system in the 1830s.[6] While in England local resistance to central direction continued to inhibit the establishment of public lunatic asylums until the 1840s, the Irish administration in Dublin was empowered to impose such institutions country-wide from 1817. What then were the pre-conditions of this power?

Foundations of the District Asylums

In the first place, it is clear that the establishment of lunatic asylums in Ireland, despite its early date, was not wholly an indigenous development. It owed much to the nature of English government in Ireland and to the contemporaneous agitation for lunacy reform in England. The latter has been well documented.

Andrew Scull, in the most critical treatment to date, has emphasised what the emergence of the public asylum in England owed to the profound social transformation wrought by capitalism. The market encouraged new distinctions between the able-bodied and the dependent unemployed: a separation which demanded a rearrangement of the institutions and mechanisms of poor relief and control. At the same time, the lunatic was coming to be seen as less brutalised and animal-like, his condition more amenable to treatment. The disruptive presence of lunatics in workhouses or gaols could be avoided by segregation in asylums where 'moral treatment', for instance, might restore reason to the lunatic.[7] Much of this analysis may apply to Ireland. But there, it must be remembered, the market was much less pervasive, its transformation of social relations throughout the

country yet to come. Indeed for many of Ireland's rulers and would-be
advisers, the problem was that the country was not yet sufficiently
capitalised. Still, while the structural effects of the development of
capitalism were less relevant in the Irish case, the ideological
responses to the changing situation in Britain made themselves felt
through the very assumptions of Ireland's rulers and leading parliamentary representatives: men like the youthful Chief Secretary,
Robert Peel, or the Waterford banker and leading Irish Whig, Sir
John Newport, who played such important roles in securing a system
of public lunatic asylums in Ireland.

English example, however, was not the only element at work in the
Irish context. What was different about Irish conditions which
prompted the foundation of a 'national' system much earlier than in
England? We need to consider three factors—the absence of a poor
law in Ireland; the scarcity of any special confinement of lunatics; and
finally the state of rural Ireland itself, its economic backwardness, the
poverty and vulnerability of its rapidly growing population, the affront
that these conditions gave to those who wished to improve Ireland and
the challenge that they offered to the maintenance of social order.

For some in both Ireland and England the absence of a poor law in
Ireland was a cause for congratulation. However that may be, it meant
that at the time of the Union Ireland was particularly devoid of
institutions and mechanisms of relief or control at a provincial or local
level. Fitful starts had been made in the eighteenth century in the
major cities, with workhouse statutes for Dublin (1703) and Cork
(1735).[8] Later in the century more decisive action was attempted in
an effort to deal with 'strolling beggars' and relief of the infirm and
aged poor. Under an Act of 1772, counties were enabled to create
corporations for the relief of the poor and for punishing vagabonds and
beggars.[9] Such corporations were empowered to establish workhouses,
or 'houses of industry', for vagrants and the destitute poor, and to
issue begging licences ('badges') to the 'deserving poor'. Certainly
this was an elementary poor law; but it lacked provision for a
compulsory rate for the establishment of workhouses. And while it
separated the 'deserving' and 'vagrant' poor in theory, it failed, as
George Nicholls (an architect of the Irish poor law) observed, to
define the distinction between the two: from the point of view of the
poor law reformers of the early nineteenth century it was therefore
quite ineffectual.[10] Nevertheless, it was through this statute that many
of the larger towns of Ireland acquired their first 'houses of industry'.
It was in these, by the end of the eighteenth century, that small

numbers of lunatics and idiots were confined. Such a development was more by default than intent, but it was administratively significant.

Specialised confinement of any sort for the insane was scarce in eighteenth-century Ireland. Apart from Dean Swift's idiosyncratic bequest for a lunatic asylum, there was evidently no other private initiative throughout the century. Swift's hospital, St Patrick's, was opened in 1757 and by 1817 had about 150 inmates: 53 fee-paying boarders and 96 paupers.[11] In a mode typical of eighteenth-century Dublin hospitals and charities it was sustained by voluntary donations and parliamentary grants. Private madhouses on the English model were rare: in 1807, when there were 45 private asylums in England, there appears to have been only one such institution in Ireland, founded in 1799 in Cork.[12] Those in Ireland able to afford it may have preferred to send lunatic relatives to English or Continental madhouses. Significantly too, the absence of a poor law requiring parishes to maintain destitute lunatics or idiots meant the absence of a market for that 'trade in lunacy' which so agitated English lunacy reformers. The expansion in numbers and size of madhouses in England was, in fact, the result of a growing tendency of parish overseers to farm out their lunatics from the workhouses to private establishments.[13] Furthermore, the small notice taken of lunatics in eighteenth-century Ireland owes something yet again to the primitive state of poor relief and its legislative appendages. It was under the laws of vagrancy that pauper lunatics and idiots had first been embraced in English statutes of 1714 and 1744.[14] Only late in the eighteenth century did the Irish legislature take note of the insane: then it was as a result of their residence in the houses of industry.

The tendency of eighteenth-century legislation was to classify and segregate the various classes of the poor. Thus, in 1772, the year of Irish workhouse legislation, another statute required the administrator of the Dublin house of industry to provide separately for the maintenance of foundlings and the control of vagrants: the presence of vagrants or beggars would be a 'bad example' (as the statute put it) to the children.[15] It was a similar logic which in 1787 provided for the separation of lunatics from the other inmates of the Irish houses of industry. Under the Prisons Act of that year, grand juries (the county administrative and judicial bodies) were empowered to establish lunatic wards in the houses of industry. These wards would house destitute idiots or insane persons, who had been certified by at least two magistrates.[16] Not only was specific provision now being made for the pauper insane: their condition was to be made the object of

inspection by the newly-created inspector-general of prisons.[17] Thus began a lengthy period during which the insane were seen anew as a class requiring separate accommodation and regulations, yet lunatics still viewed administratively as part of the wider class of the destitute poor (who required maintenance) and the criminal (who required control). At this stage their keepers did not believe their insanity remediable; provision for them did not predicate treatment and cure. This came later, in many ways as a justification for the existence of a separation which had already been achieved by institutional reform.

The third factor we must consider, one which brings us to the foundation of separate asylums, is the concern about the state of Ireland. The years after the Union were dominated politically by argument over the achievement of Catholic emancipation and about the sources of rural crime and the competence (and impartiality) of the system of justice used to control it. Frequently the two matters were seen as intermixed, becoming part of a critique of the way in which Ireland was governed and the remedies which were necessary to bring the country to tranquillity and prosperity. Thus, an attempt in 1816 by Sir John Newport to move for a parliamentary inquiry into the state of Ireland was prompted by a desire to question the government's failure to produce any measures to remedy the 'real evils' of Ireland as opposed to the heavy-handed use of insurrection acts and the maintenance of a military force to preserve the peace.[18] Any debate of this nature revolved as well around the symptoms of Ireland's condition, its relatively weak economy, blamed by such as Newport on the disabilities imposed by English policy, and its rural poverty on which Irish reformers blamed the prevalence of rural crime. Even as early as 1803, in the aftermath of the rebellion in Dublin, an Irish MP questioned the government's handling of the matter through an attempt to debate the state of Ireland and its remedies. His wide-ranging critique of the country's condition touched on the disadvantages of Catholics, absenteeism of the landlord class (itself a frequently-used justification for government intervention), and the rural poverty: 'if any doubt was entertained of the melancholy situation of Ireland, let a deputation be appointed by the House to investigate the state of the poor'.[19] As McDowell shows, the state of the poor and its remedies had been a matter of concern to Ireland's upper classes in the last turbulent decade before the Union. While Conservatives tended to deny the reality of poverty, Irish Whig interests pursued their 'programme of conciliation and reform', including 'an attempt to ameliorate the conditions of the poor'.[20] Though the state of the Irish

poor received little detailed scrutiny in the united Parliament before the 1820s, it was, however, the object of an inquiry by a select committee appointed on the motion of Newport in 1804. The emergence of the 'lunacy question' in Ireland dates in fact from this committee which found greater agreement on what to do with the insane than the sane poor. So it is from this point that we can examine the origins of the 1817 legislation for public lunatic asylums.

Inevitably Newport's committee had a broader brief than it could manage. Appointed in April 1804 it was to consider the provisions already made for the 'aged and infirm Poor of Ireland', for the punishment of vagrants and for the future care of lunatics and idiots. Not surprisingly, when it reported little more than a month later it recommended further consideration of all the subjects referred to it. Apart from its general disapproval of any adoption of a parish rate for support of the poor in Ireland, the committee's only conclusion related to the insane. The 'attention and care' (not, we may note, 'treatment') required for the relief of the lunatic and idiot could not be given to them whilst they were in a workhouse. As well, the presence of the insane in the houses of industry disrupted 'the orderly regulation of those Institutions'. The eighteenth-century legislation for houses of industry had, in any case, been ignored in most counties. Further, lunatic accommodation provided for by the 1787 Act had only been established in Dublin, Cork, Waterford and Limerick. The committee therefore recommended the establishment of four provincial lunatic asylums to be financed by the county grand juries.[21] The committee's evidence simply consisted of the returns from some counties of the provision made for the poor, together no doubt with a good dose of Newport's own arguments for a system of lunatic asylums. In his own city of Waterford, the house of industry with which he was connected had provided separate accommodation for lunatics which John Howard had praised.[22] The sources of Newport's own interest in the question of asylums are not evident from his public statements on the question. However, it is worth noting that this parliamentary initiative preceded similar moves by the English reformers by three years.[23] Indeed, Newport even pressed on with his project in 1805: a Bill for the establishment by order of the Lord-Lieutenant of four provincial asylums, each of 250 beds, was introduced in March. However, opposition to the Bill forced its withdrawal: the laws were already sufficient, opponents said, and the proposal would involve extra taxation and interference with local interests.[24]

With the failure of this premature endeavour the 'need' for separate

institutions for lunatics in Ireland was largely ignored by Parliament for another twelve years. It was within the Irish administration itself that the asylum's promoters found ready listeners. Through the Lord-Lieutenant, the Duke of Richmond, the physician and governors of the Dublin house of industry secured a government grant in 1810 for the establishment of a separate asylum for lunatics.[25] The innovation was fraught with unintended consequences. To start with, there was an ambiguity about the status of the institution—was it an asylum for the insane poor, or was it a hospital for the recovery of lunatics? The institution was already receiving patients before this question was resolved; the physician, Alexander Jackson, writing to the government in May 1814, urged that its administration should be quite distinct from that of the house of industry. Jackson made it clear that he thought of the new asylum as a 'Hospital ... instituted for the recovery of lunaticks'; its operation would be hindered by its connection with 'an institution for the reception of vagrant Beggars'.[26] For the latter the lunacy question was essentially what to do with the insane poor; for the physicians the insanity of the individual was the central issue. For representatives of Irish bourgeois urban interests, like Newport, the end in view was the effective administration of the poor; for Jackson, a member of a rising professional body whose status and reputation rested on the management of individual disabilities, the goal was the establishment of 'hospitals' free of the taint of the poorhouse.

A more immediate consequence of the government decision stemmed from the fact that the institution was declared to be, in the words of the grant, 'a general Asylum for the reception of lunatics from all parts of the kingdom'.[27] Even in 1814, Jackson could assert confidently that it would 'supersede the necessity of County Asylums'.[28] As a result the Dublin house of industry had become the major centre for the care of lunatics in Ireland between 1811 and 1815. Of 1,179 admissions to the house in those years, 754 came from outside the county and city of Dublin. From Mayo, Derry, Waterford and elsewhere, it was noted in 1817, lunatics were sent to Dublin once it became clear that they would be a continuing burden on local gaols, infirmaries or workhouses.[29] With no law of settlement in Ireland there were few barriers to foisting the poor of any county or description onto Dublin. A similar problem existed, for example, with other Dublin charitable institutions: at about this time the admission of foundlings from all over the country to the Dublin Foundling Hospital was creating enormous difficulties for that institution.[30]

The establishment of the Richmond lunatic asylum in Dublin had

therefore created not only a substantial administrative problem for its governors but also some expectations for the care of lunatics. At the same time other pressures were being brought to bear on the government. Sir John Newport, for instance, as chairman of the board of governors of the Waterford house of industry, had called for legislative provision for care of the insane poor in October 1813. Perhaps it was as a result of this appeal that in 1814 Robert Peel, as Chief Secretary for Ireland, directed an investigation of public care for lunatics.[31] In May and June 1815 the hearings of the select committee on madhouses in England presented Newport with a further opportunity to draw attention to the need for public asylums in Ireland. This appeal was supported by Edward Wakefield, prominent in the English reform movement and author of a massive statistical account of Ireland just a few years earlier. The committee took the evidence of these two, brief as it was, as definitive of the situation in Ireland: the need for public asylums was therefore declared to be even more pressing than in England.[32] At the same time as he was preparing his motion for an inquiry into the state of Ireland in April 1816, Newport again appeared before the select committee on madhouses in England, presenting in evidence his letter of 1813.[33]

At the same time, the Irish administration was being warned by its own officials of an impending accommodation crisis in the Dublin institutions. In October 1816 Peel ordered an investigation into the management of the lunatic wards of the Dublin house of industry. The report, by three army medical officers, drew attention to the widely held belief

> that buildings have lately been erected in Dublin for the reception of persons on so extensive a scale as to be able to accommodate the whole of these unhappy persons wandering over the face of the country, and inmates in gaols and hospitals.

If the government did not speedily adopt 'some humane and well-considered measures ... these miserable objects will accumulate in the capital', disturbing the Dublin institutions. The report endorsed the proposal of the Richmond asylum governors, made nearly a year previously in a letter to Peel, that facilities should be made available in Cork and Belfast for 'relief of the ... disease' outside the capital.[34] As a result Peel initiated an inquiry throughout Ireland in December 1816 to ascertain the provision for lunatics and idiots in each county. The results of this inquiry confirmed the picture painted by Newport and

others for years past. Early in the new session Peel moved for a committee to inquire into the relief of the lunatic poor in Ireland. His reasons, as he cited them in Parliament, were the pressure being placed on the Dublin institutions and the impropriety of uncontrolled lunacy: 'it was not right these unhappy beings should go abroad free from restraint'. The motion was supported by prominent English reformers, Charles Williams Wynn and George Rose, and a committee, consisting principally of Irish members, was appointed.[35] While Peel had initiated this parliamentary consideration of the question, the committee served the indispensable function of consolidating an Irish consensus for future policy, of ensuring, in fact, that legislation would proceed from the desire of Irish members rather than from the Irish executive. With a Chief Secretary like Peel, so distrustful of government intervention, one imagines this was an important consideration in the establishment of the committee.[36]

Almost exclusively the committee directed its attention to the question of where and how to provide extra accommodation for lunatics. The 'misery of madness', the 'calamity' of the insane were taken to be self-evident. The inadequacy of present arrangements was attested to by every member of the committee. It excluded the possibility of a central 'Lunatic Establishment' in Dublin which would only have confounded the difficulties already evident. The report also rejected, for reasons we will examine shortly, the option of special lunatic wards attached to county infirmaries. Instead, it was held, the 'only mode of effectual relief' would be found in the formation of district asylums 'exclusively appropriated to the reception of the insane'. In addition to the already successful asylums in Dublin and Cork, there should be established four or five asylums, of 120 to 150 beds each, in other parts of the country. Starting from the premise that it was the 'duty of the State' to provide for the 'relief and care' of lunatics, the committee recommended a substantial degree of central control. The government (that is the Lord-Lieutenant and the Privy Council) should be empowered to divide the country into suitable districts, to fix the amount of each county's contribution to the asylum, to nominate the governors and establish a board of control to oversee the system.[37] Within two weeks of the tabling of the report a Bill was drawn up embodying these recommendations and passed quickly through Parliament. Although the first asylum was begun under the auspices of this statute (57 Geo. III, c. 106) the major development of the system was undertaken after the passing of an amending Act in 1821 (1 & 2 Geo. IV, c. 33).[38] By 1835 nine asylums

were constructed in the first stage of the foundation of an asylum system in Ireland. But what was the rationale for the ready adoption by the committee of 1817 of such a substantial innovation in the field of Irish poor relief?

Two of the most forceful arguments for a system of lunatic asylums turned on the crucial issue of separation and classification. While there was some opinion in favour of lunatic cells attached to county infirmaries, two of the most vocal members of the committee vigorously opposed such a proposition. John Leslie Foster, himself a governor of the new Richmond asylum, thought it essential that 'a proper mode of treatment would be adopted and well administered' only in a few large institutions 'dedicated exclusively to that purpose'. Such a viewpoint stemmed from Foster's faith in the new system of moral treatment which, following Pinel and Tuke, was being instituted at the Richmond asylum. This system, Foster argued, required the superintendence of a 'moral governor' who exerted a total control over the management of patients.[39] The belief in the efficacy and humanity of moral treatment had brought about a significant change in attitudes to the asylum of the future in the English parliamentary inquiries of 1815-16.[40] It readily won approval from the Irish committee in 1817.

If the belief in the possibility of treatment and recovery through the special operations of the 'moral treatment' asylum was oriented primarily to the interests of the lunatic, the other argument for institutional separation looked to different interests. Thomas Spring Rice (later Lord Monteagle, a prominent figure in the Whig administrations of the 1830s) objected to the accommodation of lunatics in county infirmaries because the noise of the lunatics would destroy the repose and quiet necessary for the recuperation of infirmary cases.[41] Such an objection had long been brought against the confinement of lunatics with the sick, the poor or the criminal. Colonel Bagwell had seconded Newport's Asylums Bill in 1805 with the observation that 'the bellowing and hideous noise of the lunatics' confined in the gaol at Clonmel prevented the ordinary sick from taking their natural rest.[42] Similar preoccupations were evident in the English reform movement: the preamble to the 1808 English Asylums Act declared that the practice of confining the insane in gaols and poorhouses was 'highly dangerous and inconvenient'. This was precisely the argument of observers and managers of Irish gaols and workhouses throughout the first half of the nineteenth century. The presence of lunatics hindered the classification principle in gaols, was disruptive in workhouses and

retarded the treatment of the physically ill in infirmaries. 'The unavoidable promiscuous intercourse' with vagrants and idiots, argued the governors of the Waterford house of industry in 1816, was 'highly detrimental to the recovery of insane persons'.[43] Such views were becoming part of an orthodoxy to an age which saw opening up before it the possibilities of rehabilitation of the criminal, recovery of the lunatic and the ordinary sick, and economical relief of the poor. Thus the support of the 1817 committee for a system of lunatic asylums was founded both on a belief in the possibility of effective treatment in such institutions and on a commitment to institutional rationality, to the good order and efficient conduct of gaols, workhouses or infirmaries in which lunatics had been confined.

A further preconception of the committee, indeed of most observers of the lunacy question, was that, in addition to lunatics already confined, there were considerable numbers of insane who required suitable control. The evidence of increasing numbers of the insane in the few existing institutions inevitably fostered this impression. The necessity of providing accommodation for those not already institution- alised had varying motivations. Some reformers saw the asylums as counteracting the harsh treatment to which the insane at large were subjected. During his two years in Ireland, Edward Wakefield 'frequently saw pauper Maniacs in villages, who were the sport of the common people'.[44] Denis Browne, the Mayo MP, painted a gothic picture of madness among the peasantry with the lunatic being confined in a crib-covered hole in the floor of the cabin.[45] For such victims an asylum, whether or not it offered the chance of recovery, would be protection against the world outside. Yet other observers saw the asylum as equally offering protection to the sane. George Rose, supporting Peel's motion for an inquiry into the Irish lunatic poor in 1817, wanted to protect idiots who were 'the subject of public sport amongst children'. But he also wanted to confine maniacs who were the terror of the neighbourhood.[46] 'On most of the public roads in the South of Ireland', Crofton Croker complained in 1824, 'fools and idiots (melancholy spectacles of humanity!) are permitted to wander at large, and in consequence of this freedom have acquired vicious habits, to the annoyance of every passenger', throwing stones and so on.[47] It was this sort of image of the insane in the pre-asylum period which led the 1830 committee on the Irish poor to the view that 'wandering lunatics' had then been 'dispersed over the country in the most disgusting and wretched state'.[48]

Whether in reality the relationship of the sane and lunatic had been

quite so brutal and antagonistic is questionable. The insane were, after all, but part of a large population of beggars and vagrants in pre-Famine Ireland, a class which lived on the generosity of the cottiers and labourers. In the 1830s inquiries into the condition of the Irish poor revealed the widespread existence of this sub-culture. George Nicholls regarded the prevalence of mendicancy at the time as one of the most arresting features of the country and considered the practice to have general social support.[49] Lunatics were part of this population in receipt of popular charity. After the Famine some observers looked back, perhaps with an excessive degree of nostalgia, on the period when 'Poor Tom' always found 'a hearty welcome and a ready seat by the turf fire in the country cabin as in the comfortable farm-house'. The Famine, this writer in the Dublin *Nation* claimed, had 'destroyed the generous hospitality of the South and West'.[50] The inspectors of lunatics also noticed the impact made by the Famine on the wandering lunatics and idiots. In the Famine years, they remarked in 1864, the poor cottiers 'on whose charity their previous scanty sustenance depended' could no longer afford them relief.[51] Given the absence of a census of the insane at large in the pre-Famine period it is difficult to evaluate these observations. But to some degree, an immeasurable one, it seems that in the lunacy reformers' desire to see the insane behind the walls of an asylum—for their own or society's protection—they created an artificial problem, failing to ascertain or understand the complexity of the relationship between the 'wandering insane' and their social milieu.

Finally, in understanding the rationale behind the emergence of the asylum system in Ireland we need to explore the reasons for the ready acceptance of government direction in this area of policy. Lunatic asylums were accepted as a legitimate provision for relief of the poor with a degree of consensus which contrasts sharply with the controversy over the establishment of the Irish poor law. Already, as we have seen, Newport in 1804 had discounted the wisdom of a compulsory poor rate in Ireland while urging the necessity of public lunatic asylums. Undoubtedly the low estimate of the numbers likely to require relief meant that the financial burden of lunatic asylums would be that much less than that imposed by a poor rate.

Moreover, unlike the designers of the poor law, the makers of the new asylums were confident that the relief they were providing would not be abused. The statutes stipulated that 'all lunatic poor' within each district would be maintained in the lunatic asylum. But while the Irish poor law became notorious for restricting relief to those holding

less than a quarter-acre of land, the lunacy laws did not define the category of 'lunatic poor'.[52] Potentially at least, this gave asylums a social character different from that of workhouses. In establishing eligibility for relief, local control was exercised through the requirement of a certificate of 'poverty' issued by a clergyman or magistrate.[53] The emphasis of such a certificate was on the inability to pay for treatment in a private asylum. In administrative terms the provision for lunatics was commonly seen as part of the general area of poor relief (indeed the recommendation of the Irish poor inquiry in 1836 was that lunatic asylums should be brought under the aegis of a poor law commission)[54] but the questions were viewed by a political economist like Nassau Senior as distinct. He argued that there was no danger in the relief of calamities such as lunacy in Ireland. No public fund devoted to such relief had any tendency to diminish 'industry or providence'. Lunacy, blindness and other such disabilities were 'evils too great to allow individuals to make any sufficient provision against them, and too rare to be ... provided against by them at all'. He wanted to see an ample compulsory provision for the relief of these people.[55] A similar point was pressed on an 1830 parliamentary committee on the Irish poor by a Berkshire magistrate who had spent a summer in Ireland. Regardless of whether it had a 'tendency to lead to more misery or not' he wanted adequate relief for incurable lunatics. These people were 'the greatest objects of humane provisions'.[56] Such a view of the question owed much to a fatalist conception of the onset of lunacy—lunacy was an affliction for which neither the individual affected nor his family and immediate society was responsible. Exceptional measures for its relief and control were therefore justifiable: it was even, as the 1817 committee had asserted, the 'duty of the State' to adopt such measures. Rejecting the possibility of transferring the charge of lunatics from the county to the parish, a royal commission argued in 1858 that the existence of lunacy was 'a palpable prima facie ground for relief in the asylum, and does not call for the same scrutiny of the case' as other instances of poor relief.[57]

The humanitarian consensus was reinforced by the particular responsibilities and traditions of central government in Ireland. Dublin before the Union was, by virtue of its administrative importance and size, the location of most of Ireland's charitable institutions. Many of these were sustained by annual parliamentary grants as well as by voluntary subscription. One concession in the Act of Union was to maintain the parliamentary support of these institutions: Dublin, because of the Union, it was argued, had ceased to be a metropolis of

the wealthy but remained one of the poor. The situation of the capital, according to a parliamentary report in 1842, had only deteriorated since then. Consequently the burden of maintaining the charitable institutions had increased.[58] The implications for government involvement we have already noticed in the case of the Dublin house of industry. By acceding to the construction of a national lunatic asylum by the governors of the house of industry, the government in essence assumed responsibility for the lunatic poor of Ireland. In a climate which was admittedly congenial to such an innovation the step forward to a devolved system of lunatic asylums was easily taken.

Finally, the ease with which the government was able to impose the establishment of such a system on the counties can be attributed to the peculiar weakness of local government in Ireland. An absentee, indifferent or antagonistic gentry provided a poor basis for the reforms considered necessary in the changing conditions of the early nineteenth century. For Newport, Spring Rice and even for Peel, the failure of local authorities to provide houses of industry or lunatic accommodation under the eighteenth-century Acts meant that counties had to be forced to assume their responsibilities.[59] In England the government trod warily in directing the counties to construct asylums: the mandatory legislation followed that of Ireland by more than a quarter of a century.[60] 'Ireland', Oliver MacDonagh has suggested, 'lacked the basis for effective amateur administration.' When, in 1844, the government chose to consult the grand juries on future asylum provision Lord Monteagle warned that this would only delay needed reforms. Sending a Bill to such bodies was the worst possible course, the very reverse of action which had led to the improvement of lunatic provision under Peel.[61]

Planning, Finance and Politics

Both administrative developments and quasi-theoretical assumptions determined that Ireland would have a large number of asylums. The pre-condition for the operation of certain theoretical conceptions of planning and providing facilities for the care of the 'insane population' was, of course, the power to carry through these conceptions. The law gave such power to the central administration in Dublin. Initially this power was exercised with some restraint: at least in the first phase of asylum development (to 1835) there appears to have been little reaction on the part of local authorities to the government's plans and

directives. But the establishment in the 1840s of a department—an inspectorate within the Chief Secretary's Office—whose business was exclusively with lunatics was the origin of an unremitting struggle between Dublin and the counties over the size and financial burden of asylums. The creation of the lunatic asylums office inevitably, it seemed, meant more asylums and an increase in rates to sustain them. Indeed, the role of the inspectorate included not only the review of standards of care but the direction of the system as a whole. The tendency of such an office was to measure its achievement in terms of numbers of buildings constructed and numbers of patients accommodated. Such a tendency entailed a dangerous bureaucratic inertia which characterised the Irish lunatic asylums office later in the century. It also encouraged the continuous expansion of an institutional system which the country could ill afford.

The size and expense of the system was certainly considerable. The original system, directed in construction by an eight-member board of control appointed for the purpose alone, comprised nine asylums built at a cost of £209,000. Although each served populations of great variety in size, all the asylums were relatively small. The Waterford institution of 100 beds served the 177,000 people of the city and county of Waterford, while that at Ballinasloe, 150 beds, was the only asylum in the province of Connaught, with its population of 1,340,000.[62] For the rest, there were institutions at Armagh, Belfast and Derry in the north, Carlow and Maryborough in the midlands, Clonmel and Limerick in the south. The Richmond institution in Dublin became a district lunatic asylum in 1830 while the Cork asylum attached to the house of industry, remained outside the district system until 1845. In a second major phase of construction, this time under the inspectors of lunatic asylums, the 1850s saw new asylums at Kilkenny, Killarney, Cork, Omagh, Sligo and Mullingar as well as major new edifices at the Richmond in Dublin. Of these, only the institution at Kilkenny was of comparable size to the earlier ones, having only 152 beds. Omagh and Mullingar each had 300, while that at Cork was an imposing building capable of holding 500 inmates. In the final phase, during the 1860s, the inspectors succeeded in establishing another six district asylums at Castlebar, Downpatrick, Ennis, Enniscorthy, Letterkenny and Monaghan. In the 1860s even asylums serving only one relatively small county, like the Enniscorthy in Wexford, could be built to house 300 patients. With each new decade, then, it appeared that the authorities in Dublin considered that the country needed not only more, but larger asylums. Under these circumstances it is not

surprising to find that local authorities were questioning the government's activity in the 1850s, and even opposing its plans outright in the following decade.

The financial burden imposed on counties for all this construction was undoubtedly great. Central government advanced the capital for construction, but counties were obliged to repay these advances in fourteen years; as well they had to repay the total maintenance charges from year to year, also advanced by the Treasury. Between 1825 and 1872 the capital cost alone of the 22 asylums and land amounted to some £1,140,000.[63] The expansion as it continued into the 1860s was in striking contrast to the workhouse system. The latter was largely complete by 1850 and in apparent decline by the 1870s. The 130 workhouses built between 1839 and 1847 to accommodate 93,000 people were financed by Treasury loans totalling £1,145,000.[64] Thus comparable amounts of capital were invested in the construction of these two very different institutional systems. The scale of expenditure on lunatic asylums continued to be impressive to the end of the century; in the early 1890s loans for asylum buildings were one of the six most important loan services administered by the commissioners of public works in Ireland.[65] The outlay on the asylums is equally striking if we compare it to the institutional expenditure of the Catholic Church in Ireland in the first two-thirds of the nineteenth century. Between 1800 and 1868 almost £5,700,000 was reportedly spent on the construction of some 5,800 churches, convents, schools and other institutions.[66] By any of these standards the construction of 22 lunatic asylums and their additions entailed a substantial financial burden throughout the century.

In understanding the scope and rationale of this institutional expansion we have to turn to the activity and mentality of the inspectors of lunatics. The establishment of a special inspectorate is examined in another context.[67] Here we need only note that by the 1850s the inspectors were the effective administrators of the whole system. Under the Act appointing them, reported a royal commission in 1858, the inspectors

> have practically undertaken most, if not all the duties, connected with the superintendence of and direction of asylums ... in fact all matters relating to them are now submitted to their consideration by the Executive, which relies upon them in regard to the formation of new districts, the localities where the asylums should be erected, and the extent of their accommodation.[68]

Consequently, while the original size of the asylum system, as seen by the 1817 committee and the board of control in the 1820s and 1830s, had been quite limited in both numbers of asylums and bed size, by the middle of the century new assumptions were operative.

The first concerned the numbers of inmates. Already by the early 1840s it was becoming clear that the new asylums were overcrowded. In 1843 a parliamentary committee reported that the asylums now contained 2,028 inmates although they had been built for only 1,220. The major problem was that the number of incurable inmates was rapidly increasing, diminishing the efficacy of these 'Hospitals for the Cure of Insanity'. The committee recommended a general expansion of asylum accommodation while remaining non-committal on the problem of housing 'incurables'.[69] One suggestion, even embodied in a statute in 1845, was to establish special, more economical, asylums for incurables. Francis White, the first inspector of lunatics, was initially in favour of such institutions: 'Asylums for the chronic insane classes', as he styled them, as opposed to the 'Hospitals for the treatment of Insanity'.[70] After only a year in his new position, however, he opposed the idea of separation. It was difficult to decide who was curable and who incurable and, like John Conolly (the English specialist who had given evidence to the 1843 committee), he felt that an 'incurables asylum' would have a bad effect on the inmates, only confirming their hopelessness.[71] Administratively difficult as any other decision might have been, this decision to maintain the 'chronic classes' inevitably meant more and larger asylums. Ten years later its implications were well understood: in 1856 the Donegal grand jury protested against the opening of lunatic asylums for harmless idiots, epileptics, imbeciles and lunatics, which involved institutional expansion and greater taxation, the latter perhaps potentially exceeding the total amounts being levied for poor relief and medical charities.[72]

The inspectorate's acceptance of the continuing presence of the incurable pointed to the need for more asylum beds. But no one knew how to estimate the right number. White was concerned to establish what insane population outside the asylum was likely to require future accommodation. The 1841 Irish census had included a count of the insane but this was deficient because it did not record those at large.[73] So it was probably at White's instance that the Chief Secretary's Office ordered a census of the insane at large to be made by the constabulary. In 1844 the police estimated that there were 6,217 'harmless Idiots and Simpletons' not in institutions. In White's report

on the future needs of the asylum system this statistic was translated into 6,217 wandering lunatics and idiots 'amongst whom instances frequently occur of violence and mania, which demand immediate attention, as they become both dangerous to themselves and the community'. He believed that from 'such a mass of afflicted beings many will be found hereafter fit claimants for the humane and charitable bounty of the public, and will add considerably to the numbers already in the Asylums'.[74] For White, asylum statistics were not the best data on which to estimate 'the relative proportion of insanity in each district'.[75] Hence statistics of the insane at large, which indicated a much greater problem than originally conceived, were considered highly relevant. Over the next fifteen years there was a plethora of such surveys: again by the police (extending to a record of the personal details, name, age, address and religion of all insane not in institutions), as well as by the poor law commissioners and the census commissioners.[76]

While the value of such surveys was viewed with increasing scepticism from the later 1850s[77] their significance lay quite outside the question of their accuracy or their assumptions. They created an expectation of a relatively large lunatic population which might require institutional care in the future. In failing to take account of 'new' cases of insanity in the community of the sane the surveys were also fated to be illusory: even if all the recognised insane could be housed, each year would bring forward yet more cases of recent origin. The inspectors were not unaware of the latter problem but contemporary estimates of the incidence of insanity in the community were quite primitive. They were usually guesses, or else referred to quite varied populations, and were based on current asylum populations as a proportion of the community (that is a prevalence rate, with little predictive value for planning purposes). The poverty of the measures available was exemplified in the estimation of the needs of the Dublin district. The commissioners of public works had arrived at a projection of extra accommodation for 460 pauper lunatics by taking the 'pauper population' of the Dublin district for 1841 and assuming from English figures a lunacy rate of one in every thousand. They also expected (in January 1848) that there would be some improvement in the condition of the poor, with a consequent easing of future demand. The inspectors, on the other hand, regarded the commissioners' calculations as far too low and pointed out that the English commissioners in lunacy had considered their own estimate was well short of the real rate of lunacy. Moreover, they believed, the conditions of a metropolis

were more conducive to madness than elsewhere.[78] It was on the basis
of these crude statistics and assumptions that the lunacy authorities
attempted to calculate the future needs of the community. In the end,
of course, it was the local community which would determine the
patterns of use of these institutions and which had to pay for them.

The siting of asylums could bring both benefits and disadvantages
to a locality. Consequently local reaction to the decisions taken in
Dublin were varied, sometimes even contradictory. In the 1840s in
particular the immediate economic advantages of having a major
institution constructed in a provincial town made an asylum desirable.
The grand jury of the North Riding of Tipperary, for example, urged
the Lord-Lieutenant to locate an asylum for incurable lunatics from
the province of Munster in Nenagh: as well as the usual arguments
proffered in such a petition—the situation, the centrality of the town, a
well-motivated local gentry who could provide an active governing
board—the petition cited the ready access of the town to provisions
and fuel.[79] An asylum offered not only the attraction of employment
opportunities during construction and in its everyday operation, but
contracts for stores, fuel and so on. During the Famine in particular
the employment offered by the construction of a new asylum pressed
more than one town to urge the government to finance asylum works
immediately. The Limerick asylum board agreed to the separation of
Kerry from the district in May 1846, calling for the speedy commence-
ment of work on a Killarney asylum in order to extend 'employment
to the destitute poor at this pressing emergency'.[80] In 1848, following
threats of violence from the poor of Sligo and Kilkenny, the mayors of
both towns called on the government to start work on the planned
asylums.[81]

The support for new asylums was thus fostered at a local level by
considerations additional to the problem of accommodating the
insane. Taxation was yet another factor. The three or four component
counties of large districts inevitably wrangled about their share of the
asylum's services and costs. Lord Westmeath complained in 1844
that the county of Westmeath derived little benefit from the district
asylum in Maryborough. The placing of the asylum in that town had
been, he said, a 'great job in favour of the Queen's County'.[82] In 1845
the Fermanagh grand jury complained that a fair proportion of the
county's lunatics were not being admitted to the Armagh asylum.
Three years later it protested that the placing of the new district
asylum in Omagh (Co. Tyrone) would still leave it out of the direct
control of Fermanagh. Similar arguments led the Wexford grand jury

in 1856 to the demand for a separate asylum for the county alone.[83]

It was in this context that the inspector of lunatics prepared for the construction of six new district asylums from 1849. Instructions issued by the board of works required the architects to remember that they were designing 'an hospital and not a prison'. A 'Gothic' style was recommended, the interiors to be lined with bricks but unplastered, the wards to be classified from ground up, according to the degree of refractoriness of the patients, a warm bath, water closet and washing room to be provided in each ward, and the asylum to include an infirmary and a chapel.[84] The resulting institutions were sober and imposing in their presence, usually located on the outskirts of the major town of the district, close enough to services, but rural enough to have at least a few acres of farming land.

While the government had been able to embark on this trebling of asylum accommodation with little controversy, by the mid-1850s local enthusiasm had waned. Already the inspectors were forced to defend the great size of the new asylums in 1852: the insane 'tended to accumulate' and the population of many districts had been much greater a few years before.[85] In 1854 a number of counties protested to the Chancellor of the Exchequer about the high cost and imperfect work in some asylums. A subsequent Treasury inquiry and a parliamentary select committee both found that local authorities were justified in complaining about the way Dublin had directed the work. The first round of construction before 1835 had been directed by a specially appointed board of control which laid estimates before the grand juries prior to construction. This consultation was absent under the inspectors, who directed proceedings from Dublin and whose poor communication with the board of works had even resulted in irregularities in the issuing of advances from the Treasury.[86] The government was forced to legislate to regularise the repayment of the Treasury advances and to remit some payments where asylums had been badly constructed or extravagantly decorated.[87]

Bureaucratic centralism came under fire yet again in the 1850s in the matter of asylum appointments. From 1843, Privy Council 'rules and regulations for lunatic asylums' had required an establishment including chaplains in each asylum. While most asylum boards had appointed chaplains representing the denominations, those at Belfast and Armagh did not. Religious divisions in the Presbyterian community in Belfast appear to have been crucial in this decision.[88] In 1853, however, the government decided to force the Belfast board's hand by appointing chaplains and requiring the board to pay them salaries. In

subsequent legal action the High Court found that appointments made by the Lord-Lieutenant were illegal since he had 'personally' appointed them without statutory authority.[89] The previously unchallenged authority of the Lord-Lieutenant (and, of course, the inspectorate) was shaken by the decision. The government was forced to review its rights of appointment (or 'patronage' as it was almost invariably referred to) and in fact the whole question of its direction of lunatic asylums.

At Dublin Castle the Under-Secretary, Thomas Larcom, had already been considering devolving control of the lunatic asylums in the light of the 'unpleasant collisons' over repayments and appointments. Since the 'necessity for these Hospitals [was now] universally admitted' he believed that the grand juries and the boards of governors could safely be given responsibility for them with the government merely ensuring the maintenance of standards through the inspectorate. However, the Chief Secretary at the time, Edward Horsman, was wary of such an 'experiment'.[90] Consequently, the first attempt by the government to regularise the control of asylums following the High Court judgement was on centralist lines. It was also a blunder. Having wrongly assumed that all appointments in the past had been made by the Lord-Lieutenant, the government introduced a Bill which validated all previous appointments and vested future ones in the Irish executive. There was an outcry from Irish members over what Horsman himself described as this 'wholesale invasion of patronage rights' and the Bill was defeated.[91] The government then appointed a royal commission, ostensibly to investigate the conditions of Irish asylums which had been criticised privately by the Treasury commissioners of inquiry;[92] but in fact the royal commission was an attempt to find a new meeting ground between the centralist desire to regulate asylum standards and the local demand for autonomous management.

While uncovering much evidence about the day-to-day operation of the Irish asylums the royal commission's impact was minimal. The English model of administration was its principal recommendation: a central board of commissioners for lunacy which would stand in relation to the boards of governors in much the same way as the poor law commissioners to the guardians. That is, the central board would set minimum standards and, if necessary, compel governors to meet them. The governors would, in the majority, be appointed by the grand juries. They would be empowered to appoint the physician and other senior officers.[93] Yet when the new Conservative Chief Secretary,

Lord Naas, came to enact this increase in local control in 1859 he was soundly defeated. Catholic interests were dissatisfied with a transfer of control to the largely Protestant grand juries, and one inspector of lunatics himself lobbied actively against the changes because, Naas believed, he had wanted a commission in lunacy rather than just an inspectorate.[94] Legislative change having failed, the government fell back on the rather unsatisfactory *status quo*. The position of the inspectors was effectively maintained, indeed even improved: in 1860, together with two officials from the board of works, they were appointed to a board of control for the construction of asylums. Under this body a further six asylums were established in the following decade. New Privy Council rules and regulations in 1862 added to the inspectors' powers of intervention in asylum matters, such as dietary standards and stores' contracts.[95] At the same time memories of the reaction to Dublin's heavy-handedness in the early 1850s made the Irish executive more conciliatory to local interests. It was not until late in the decade that the Belfast chaplaincy question was resolved by legislation forcing the asylum board to appoint chaplains.[96] And in spite of the interventionist advice of his bureaucratic advisers, the Chief Secretary, Sir Robert Peel, did not resort to the use of the government's legal powers to establish new asylums in Louth and Wicklow.[97] Nevertheless, however tense the relationship of Dublin Castle to local government may have been in the 1850s and 1860s, asylum expansion was remarkable: the 2,802 beds in the district asylums in 1851 had grown to 4,623 in 1861 and 7,831 in 1871. At the same time as the two tiers of government were contending for external control, another set of politics was determining the character of internal management of the asylum.

From Moral Governors to Medical Superintendents

The early asylums, inspired as they were by the ideology of moral treatment, were managed not by medical men but by laymen. The 'superior resident officer' of the district asylum in the 1820s and 1830s was the 'Moral Governor', responsible to the asylum board alone. The business of an asylum was taken to be management and guidance of the patient, not his subjection to physical treatment. Thus the moral governor of the Richmond asylum was required to

make himself acquainted with the cases of the patients, and to

maintain intercourse with them, so as to be able to report to the Visitors appointed by the Board the character of their derangement and the observations he has made on the mode of moral management or style of conversation which seems best adapted to supply motives of self-restraint, or to repress the instance of frantic paroxysms.

There was nothing in the training of a physician or apothecary which especially qualified him for these duties.[98] For the most part then, non-medical appointments were made to these positions. Yet where medically-qualified men were appointed (in particular, Robert Stewart, an apothecary, to Belfast in 1835, and James Flynn, a physician, to Clonmel in 1841), they worked energetically to create an asylum system dominated by medical men. Potential for subversion of the lay managers' position also developed in the appointment to all asylums of visiting physicians. The rationale for such appointments was treatment of the patient's physical illness where any existed. However, already by 1835 it was clear to the medical investigators of the Irish poor inquiry that there was no uniformity in the systems of management in Irish lunatic asylums. They contrasted the 'moral treatment' system at Carlow asylum with the medical system at Maryborough (where 41 patients were taking medicines for the 'cure' of insanity) and found the results comparable. In fact, while the lay 'moral governor' at Carlow had retained his control of the institution, at Maryborough a particularly forceful physician, Dr John Jacob, had succeeded in establishing his authority over the lay manager in aspects of treatment of patients: the manager there, the royal commission investigator reported, was no more than an 'upper keeper'.[99] Consequently, within only a few years of their opening, Irish asylums of the late 1830s were showing some signs of a substantial change in their domestic management.

That change revolved around the interests of the increasingly self-confident medical profession. In England the medical men had weathered the considerable blow to their reputation dealt out by the parliamentary inquiries into madhouses and the medical treatment of the insane. Scull has shown how successfully the physicians fought to regain the ground they had lost: on both a central legislative level and on the local level the physicians succeeded by the 1830s in establishing medical control of asylum management, and even in substantially influencing the inspection system.[100] In Ireland the story was essentially the same though the crucial developments took place at a later stage;

later, because there was little professional involvement with lunatic asylums of any description before the emergence of the district asylums. There too the aspiring asylum superintendents advanced claims for their authority on the grounds of an expertise which was patently non-existent. And having an organisational and political capacity which far exceeded that of the lay managers who had none, establishment of medical hegemony was easily accomplished. While, as we have seen, the basis for a medical take-over was already emerging in a number of asylums in the 1830s, it was in Dublin Castle that the attainment of medical control was ensured through the foundation of a lunacy inspectorate.

The separation of the inspection of asylums from that of prisons was largely the product of one man's activity. Francis White, surgeon to the Richmond asylum since 1835, previously secretary to the board of health during the cholera epidemic of 1832, was the first to question the adequacy of the inspection system in 1841. Since 1787 the inspector of prisons in Ireland had been responsible for inspecting asylums: with the establishment of district asylums the two inspectors-general of prisons, Majors Woodward and Palmer, were directed to inspect asylums as well.[101] Their activities and responsibilities in this area, however, were relatively passive and in 1841 White launched an attack on the inspection system. In a letter to a commission inquiring into the grand jury laws in Ireland he claimed that the inspection of asylums was without any 'beneficial result'. The period of inspection was known beforehand and limited to minor matters in any case. It was a duty totally unconnected with the inspectorship of prisons, he asserted, and would remain deficient until it

> be made by persons who will be able to afford more time towards the performance of such important duties, and who should possess that species of knowledge which is necessary, and which cannot be possessed by those whose education and previous habits have not qualified them for the peculiar duty in question.[102]

This criticism, embodying an undisguised plea for the appointment of medical inspectors of asylums, was accepted without question by the commissioners who duly criticised the efficiency of the prisons' inspectors. Instead, the commission report recommended the transfer of the inspection to the poor law commissioners, in line with its proposed transfer of lunatic charges to the poor rates.[103] White's letter, on the other hand, had brought him to notice and, when Major

Woodward died later in the year, he was appointed an inspector of prisons. From this position, which he occupied for four years, he worked to establish a separate lunacy inspectorate.

In the person of a new Lord Chancellor, Sir Edward Sugden, White's plans to reconstitute asylum administration found ready acceptance. Only a year after his appointment a major piece of legislation was enacted making the inspectors of prisons also inspectors of lunatic asylums.[104] From this point on White appeared to be playing a major role in the administration of asylums. As adviser to Sugden he played the greater part in the drafting of the first Privy Council rules for the regulation of district asylums, ordered in 1843.[105] In the same year he was a major witness before a House of Lords select committee on the state of the lunatic poor in Ireland. Although the committee had been formed on the motion of Lord Monteagle, who was convinced of the worth of moral treatment and not partial to the necessity of medical influence in asylums, White used the occasion to press the priority of medical claims. Not surprisingly then, the committee supported a lunacy inspectorate separate from that for prisons. Inspection of asylums was assumed in this report to be more intimately connected with that of medical services.[106] The committee's recommendation for more asylum accommodation provided further opportunity for White's initiatives. In 1844 he was actively engaged in reporting to the government on the future scope of the asylum system, as we have seen earlier. In August of the following year, just four years after his appointment to the prisons' inspectorate, legislation empowered the Lord-Lieutenant to appoint one or two inspectors of lunatics who were to assume all functions of the inspectors of prisons relating to lunatics.[107] Francis White was the inevitable choice for the first appointment to the new post on 1 January 1846. The legislation said nothing about the qualifications necessary for the post but from the beginning in Ireland it was assumed that only doctors would be appointed. Such was the consensus for medical expertise in the management of the insane. In England the survival of an older prejudice against the doctors ensured that still only half the commissioners in lunacy, counterparts to the Irish inspectors, were medical men. Yet when the second inspector was appointed in Ireland in 1847 it was again a doctor, John Nugent, who had been travelling physician to Daniel O'Connell.[108] Between them the two medical men ensured by 1870 that the asylums were removed from lay management or surveillance.

The crucial step in this process was the standardisation of asylum

regulations in 1843. White had been largely responsible for the Privy Council rules ordered in that year. Such rules were necessary, as he explained to the 1843 committee on the lunatic poor, because the asylums had not fulfilled their object of cure in spite of their great cost. Implying that the absence of medical management was to blame for this failure he argued that what was needed was a set of rules which would define the duties of various officers in the asylums. When Sugden agreed to establish a uniform set of rules White drafted them without communicating with any asylum personnel, with the crucial exception, as he admitted, of 'some of the Medical Officers'.[109] Consequently, the rules proved to be a complete reversal of previous responsibilities in the asylum. The visiting physician was entrusted with complete responsibility for the *moral* as well as medical treatment of the inmates. The manager (even if a medical man, as at Belfast and Clonmel) was now merely the agent of the physician in respect of treatment.[110]

The reaction to the rules made it clear that White had not resolved the question of *which* medical men should control the asylum. White was probably more partial to the interests of the visiting physicians, frequently men of some standing in their profession and in the community, than of the medical managers. At Belfast, for instance, the board had appointed Robert Stewart, an apothecary, as the resident manager. White conceded that the managers themselves felt 'slighted and thrown in the Shade by [the rules]' but was confident that, upon 'mature consideration', the Lords committee would conclude that the new arrangements were advantageous to 'Public and Patient'. The possibility of any other opinion on the matter was dismissed with an appeal to the authority of his profession. Major Woodward, whom White had succeeded as inspector of prisons, had objected to medical control but, of course, 'not being a Medical Man [he] could not be held to have the best Experience in such Matters'.[111] The boast of medical expertise was the basis for the profession's claim to the management of asylums. 'Medical Science', A.R. Blake told the 1843 committee, was necessary to the proper functioning of the asylum.[112] The chairman of the contemporaneous select committee on medical charities in Ireland clearly considered that the classification of inmates and the recording of changes in the patient required 'the services of a scientific and well-educated individual'. Another member of that committee recommended the English practice of appointing medical managers as good policy for Ireland.[113] Rare were those like Monteagle who still in 1843 disagreed with the proposition that the

'moral Governor' of an asylum should have 'Medical Knowledge as a necessary Qualification'.[114] The consensus for medical control was overwhelming. Within the profession, however, the 1843 rules created a division of interests and opportunities. The future lay, not with the visiting physicians, but with the medical managers who were soon calling themselves resident physicians.

If men like Flynn and Stewart were effectively to challenge the newly-won authority of the visiting physicians it was important to have *medical* managers in other district asylums. This was increasingly the case since the inspectors of lunatics promoted the practice from the start of their appointment. 'Public opinion', they claimed in their report for 1846, was now generally favourable to medical managers.[115] Medical journals advocated the appointment of resident physicians. Robert Stewart was probably the anonymous reviewer of lunacy reports who constantly advocated the innovation in the pages of the re-established *Dublin Journal of Medical Science* from 1846.[116] In its first number Forbes Winslow's *Journal of Psychological Medicine* criticised the absence of resident physicians in Irish asylums. Winslow argued that restraint and ill-treatment were unavoidable in the absence of a medical officer; the visiting physician system encouraged irregular medical attendance and was disruptive to the institution.[117] With the retirement of the older managers and the opening of new asylums in the early 1850s the inspectors were able to do what 'public opinion' wanted and appoint doctors as managers. The *Dublin Journal of Medical Science* welcomed the appointment of a doctor to Carlow in 1850 and suggested that the title 'manager' be discontinued since physicians were being appointed; 'Hospitals for the Insane' should similarly be substituted for 'Lunatic Asylums'.[118] By 1858 the practice was so generally accepted that the royal commission into lunatic asylums considered that new regulations were required to take account of the medical officers who were managers—they should, for instance, be disqualified from private practice.[119] Such a suggestion implied that medical managers should devote themselves exclusively to asylum management and the treatment of the insane, a short step indeed from the identification of asylum work as in itself a medical speciality. The 'resident physicians' were already working to elevate their work in this way.

From the early 1840s an Association of Medical Officers of Hospitals for the Insane was formed in England, meeting intermittently to consider common interests.[120] When the association began to act more purposefully in 1851 Robert Stewart was involved as the only

Irish doctor present at the annual meeting in July.[121] As more doctors became asylum managers they joined the association: men like Joseph Lalor who had been physician to the old Kilkenny asylum before being appointed as the first resident physician to the Richmond in Dublin. The English and Scottish members of the association were eager to support their Irish colleagues in first lobbying for the appointment of medical men in *all* public asylums and then in their struggle against the authority of the non-resident physicians. Professional opportunity and social status were both at stake in this campaign. In seconding a motion that the Irish government should appoint only medical officers as managers, an English doctor urged the association to avail itself

> of every opportunity to show the government and the public that lunacy is the result of disease. Unfortunately, an opinion was too prevalent that lunacy is out of the category of the disease; and they found as a consequence, that medical men were degraded to the point of mere keepers of mad houses.

This 'degradation' even extended to a financial undervaluation of the doctor's services, to his being paid the same salary as his lay predecessor. When in 1851 the inspectors of lunatics recommended better salaries for the medical superintendents it was probably the pen of Robert Stewart which commended their action in the pages of the *Dublin Journal of Medical Science*. The non-professional managers had rendered minor services compared to that offered by medical men and were of a 'different grade altogether in the social scale to the present superintendents': the present salary of two hundred pounds was 'barely sufficient to enable them to keep up the appearance of gentlemen'.[122]

With the support of their British colleagues the Irish asylum physicians pressed their professional claims forcefully from 1860. Joseph Lalor of the Richmond asylum published a pamphlet which urged the appointment of more medical staff in Irish asylums and the total care of inmates by resident staff. The *Dublin Medical Press*, which defended the place of the non-resident physician in the asylum hierarchy, castigated Lalor's tract but it received wholesome praise from John Bucknill, the prominent English alienist and editor of the *Journal of Medical Science*.[123] At the annual meeting of the association shortly afterwards Lalor was elected president for 1861; the annual meeting for that year would be held in Dublin, a move

advocated by Dr Flynn of Clonmel on the grounds that it would do much to promote the position of resident medical officers in Irish asylums. The association further resolved, on the motion of John Conolly, that the management of asylums and treatment of patients should be given to resident physicians, leaving the non-resident merely in the position of consultant.[124]

The basis for the alienists' claim to expertise was purely experiential. Neither they nor the non-resident physicians could claim any special training in 'mental diseases' before the 1870s. Instead the alienists used their constant attendance on the insane as the evidence of their expertise. Theirs was a neater and more logical position than that taken by the visiting physicians. If medical treatment was necessary (there was by now no dispute about this) then constant medical superintendence was surely essential: the capacity to do this only derived from years of continuing contact with the insane. To the opposition of Dominic Corrigan, president of the Irish College of Physicians and one of the royal commissioners in 1858, the medical superintendents responded with the jibe that 'however high his reputation in other branches of the profession [he] had so few opportunities of acquiring a knowledge of this'.[125]

By this stage there was probably no need to argue the case. The position of the non-resident physicians was largely anachronistic with the disappearance of the lay managers. Dublin Castle certainly thought so. In 1860 a dispute between Dr Jacob, the Maryborough physician, and Dr Burton, the asylum manager, gave Inspector Nugent the opportunity to urge the revision of the 1843 rules. When Dr Jacob appealed to the Privy Council rules as authority for his superintendence of medical treatment, Nugent responded bluntly that the rules are 'quite as well in some respects avoided'. He impressed on the asylum board that the 'Inspectors and the Government are far from thinking that the rules and regulations laid down by the Privy Council are proper'.[126] Then, just two weeks before the 1861 annual meeting of the alienists in Dublin, a Waterford MP, J.A. Blake, delivered an attack on the management of the insane in Irish asylums. In part this was a criticism of asylum facilities, drawing on evidence from the royal commission's report. But included was a strong plea for the advancement of the status of the medical managers: he wanted inspectors who had previous experience of the treatment of insanity, that is asylum doctors, as well as the total management of asylums by resident medical officers. Whether Blake's move was timed to coincide with the association's Dublin meeting is unclear but signifi-

cantly the Waterford asylum, of which he was a governor, was the last in Ireland to have a lay manager.[127] A deputation from the association, meeting under Lalor's presidency, presented their case to an evidently sympathetic Sir Robert Peel. Consequently a complete revision of the 1843 rules was carried out in 1862 in spite of some public opposition and even resistance on the Privy Council.[128]

The 1862 rules established conclusively the authority of the 'resident medical superintendent' in the asylum. A qualified physician and surgeon, he was to be responsible for the medical and moral treatment of all patients and for the domestic management of the asylum. The 'visiting physician', as the rules denominated him, had in fact only a consulting role, being called in by the superintendent as he thought fit and 'visiting' only with the latter's consent.[129] This thorough victory for the asylum doctors ensured of course not only their own security in a well-rewarded position of authority; it was equally the condition for the emergence, as elsewhere, of a new specialisation in medicine, that of psychiatry. Its emergence was determined not by a theoretical or empirical advance but by institutional politics.

There was another major consequence of the 1862 rules. The negative face of the rise of the asylum doctor was the decline of lay interest and involvement in the lunacy question. J.A. Blake continued to urge improvements in 'moral treatment' in Irish asylums throughout the 1860s but this appeal was now rather idiosyncratic. From the beginning of the century to the 1840s the activity of lay reformers had been central to the restructuring of institutional care of lunatics in Britain and Ireland. By the 1860s these reformers were mostly dead or, like Shaftesbury, wholly converted to the primacy of medical intervention and control. By handing over asylums to doctors, governments had, to a great extent, removed the institutions and their inmates from the public arena. It was not until the Edwardian era (and then only to a limited extent in Ireland) that insanity again came under public scrutiny in a serious way. In the meantime the *status quo* was only occasionally threatened by public dismay at the increasing financial burden of the asylums or by administrative ineptitude and stagnation.

Notes

1. Gearóid Ó'Tuathaigh, *Ireland before the Famine 1798-1848* (Gill and Macmillan, Dublin, 1972), p. 115. For the state's activity in Ireland in this period, see ibid., pp. 80-

116; Oliver MacDonagh, *Ireland: The Union and its Aftermath* (Allen and Unwin, London, 1977), pp. 33-52, and *Early Victorian Government 1830-1870* (Weidenfeld and Nicolson, London, 1977), pp. 178-96. R.B. McDowell, *Public Opinion and Government Policy in Ireland, 1801-1846* (Faber, London, 1952) and R.D.C. Black, *Economic Thought and the Irish Question: 1817-1870* (Cambridge University Press, Cambridge, 1960) provide much of the political and ideological context for government activity in Ireland at this time.

2. Cf. Black, *Economic Thought and the Irish Question*, pp. 105-12, 190-4.

3. W.M. Thackeray, *The Irish Sketch Book*, in *The Biographical Edition of the Works of William Makepeace Thackeray*, Vol. 5 (Smith, Elder, London, 1898), p. 571.

4. Sir Francis Bond Head, *A Fortnight in Ireland* (1852), p. 179 for his visit to the Clifden workhouse: 'as I only wanted to see its inmates, I requested the master to assemble them, at once, in their respective yards'.

5. H. Martineau, *Letters from Ireland* (John Murray, London, 1853), p. 170.

6. D. Akenson, *The Irish Education Experiment* (Routledge, London, 1970), pp. 17-19. On the structure of government in Ireland under the Union see R.B. McDowell, *The Irish Administration 1801-1914* (Routledge, London, 1964).

7. Andrew T. Scull, *Museums of Madness: The Social Organization of Insanity in Nineteenth-Century England* (Allen Lane, London, 1979), chs. 1 and 2.

8. G. Nicholls, *A History of the Irish Poor Law* (London, 1856), pp. 35-42.

9. 11 & 12 Geo. III (Ire.), c.30; see Nicholls, *History of the Irish Poor Law,* pp.51-7.

10. Ibid., p. 56.

11. *Select Committee on the Lunatic Poor in Ireland*, p. 46, *HC* (1817), viii, hereafter cited as *Lunatic Poor*.

12. W.Ll. Parry-Jones, *The Trade in Lunacy* (Routledge, London, 1972), p. 30; Arthur Williamson, 'The Beginnings of State Care for the Mentally Ill in Ireland', *Economic and Social Review*, vol. 1, no. 2 (1970), p. 285.

13. Cf. Scull, *Museums of Madness*, pp. 50-4 and Parry-Jones, *The Trade in Lunacy*, pp. 9-14. The law in England did not require licensing or inspection of houses in which *pauper* lunatics were kept.

14. 12 Anne (II), c. 23 and 17 Geo. II, c. 5. See K. Jones, *A History of the Mental Health Services* (Routledge, London, 1972), pp. 25-8.

15. Nicholls, *History of the Irish Poor Law*, p. 46.

16. 27 Geo. III (Ire.), c. 39, s. 8. A later Act (46 Geo. III, c. 95) increased the amounts grand juries could raise for this purpose.

17. 27 Geo. III (Ire.), c. 39, s. 12.

18. *Hansard*, lst ser., vol. 34, 11-24 (26 April 1816).

19. *The Parliamentary History of England from the earliest period to the year 1803* (London, 1820), vol. xxxvi, p. 1703 (Mr Hutchinson, 11 August 1803).

20. R.B. McDowell, *Irish Public Opinion 1750-1800* (Faber, London, 1944), pp. 229-32.

21. *Report from the Committee appointed to consider the ... provisions for the care of Lunatics and Idiots by Grand Jury Presentments, HC* (1803-4), iv.

22. *Hansard*, 1st ser., vol. 4, 206 (4 April 1805). The institution's conditions were less praiseworthy in 1816, cf. *Lunatic Poor*, pp. 40-42.

23. Cf. Jones, *History of the Mental Health Services*, pp. 57-61.

24. *Hansard*, 1st ser., vol. 4, 206-7 (4 April 1805).

25. Cf. A.P. Williamson, 'The Origins of the Irish Mental Hospital Service, 1800-1843', M Litt thesis, Trinity College, Dublin, 1970, pp. 43-7, 101-2.

26. Letter of Alexander Jackson, 30 May 1814, Peel Papers, British Museum Additional MS. 40236, 132/3.

27. *Journal of the House of Commons*, vol. 65 (1810), p. 589.

28. See note 25.

29. *Lunatic Poor*, pp. 7, 9, 11, 34.

30. K.H. Connell, *Irish Peasant Society* (Clarendon Press, Oxford, 1968), pp. 72-3.

31. Cf. Williamson, 'Beginnings of State Care for the Mentally Ill in Ireland', pp. 282-3. See *First Report. Minutes of Evidence taken before the Select Committee ... for the better Regulation of Madhouses in England*, p. 94, *HC* (1816), vi, for Newport's letter of 1813.

32. *Report from the Committee on Madhouses in England*, p. 4, *HC* (1814-15), iv. On the committee, see Scull, *Museums of Madness*, pp. 76-82.

33. See note 31.

34. *Lunatic Poor*, pp. 28-30.

35. *Hansard*, 1st ser., vol. 35, 881-3 (4 March 1817).

36. Cf. McDowell, *Public Opinion and Government Policy in Ireland*, pp. 70-1, 211-12.

37. *Lunatic Poor*, p. 4.

38. *Journal of the House of Commons*, vol. 72 (1817); Williamson, 'Beginnings of State Care for the Mentally Ill in Ireland', p. 286.

39. *Lunatic Poor*, pp. 10-11.

40. Cf. Scull, *Museums of Madness*, pp. 68-70.

41. *Lunatic Poor*, p. 21.

42. *Hansard*, 1st ser., vol. 4, 66-7 (21 March 1805).

43. *Lunatic Poor*, p. 39; for an articulation of this view in the 1840s see the speeches of Lord Monteagle on the confinement of lunatics in Irish gaols: *Hansard*, 3rd ser., vol. 68 (25 April 1843) and vol. 76 (11 July 1844). In 1845 the Chief Secretary, Sir Thomas Fremantle, legislated for the establishment of a central asylum for criminal lunatics (the Dundrum asylum in Dublin) on the grounds that it was 'inexpedient to confine criminal lunatics in gaols and other places'. *Hansard*, 3rd ser., vol. 80, 586 (19 May 1845).

44. *First Report. Minutes of Evidence taken before the Select Committee on Madhouses in England*, p. 24, *HC* (1814-15), iv.

45. *Lunatic Poor*, p. 23, Cf. Williamson, 'Beginnings of State Care for the Mentally Ill in Ireland', pp. 283-4.

46. *Hansard*, 1st ser., vol. 35, 881-3 (4 March 1817).

47. T. Crofton Croker, *Researches in the South of Ireland* (1824), Shannon (Irish University Press, Shannon, 1969), p. 35.

48. *Report of the Select Committee on the State of the Poor in Ireland*, p. 28, *HC* (1830), vii.

49. Cf. Nicholls, *History of the Irish Poor Law*, p. 182. The evidence relating to 'Vagrancy' is in the *First Report. Royal Commission into the Condition of the Poorer Classes in Ireland Appendix (A)*, pp. 475-793, *HC* (1835), xxxii.

50. *Nation*, 1 October 1859, press cutting in Larcom Papers, NLI, MS. 7776.

51. *14th Report on the District, Local and Private Lunatic Asylums in Ireland*, p. 18, *HC* (1865), xxi (hereafter these annual reports cited as '*14th Report*', etc.).

52. Black, *Economic Thought and the Irish Question*, pp. 125-6; the effect of the Gregory clause 'was to prevent any person holding more than a quarter-acre of land from receiving relief until he had parted with possession of the land'.

53. For forms of admission to Cork, Sligo and Waterford see *Report of the Commissioners of Inquiry into the ... Treatment of the Insane in Ireland*, pp. 128-30, *HC* (1857-8), xxvii (hereafter *Royal Commission*).

54. Cf. McDowell, *Public Opinion and Government Policy*, p. 192 for a summary of the commissioners' recommendations.

55. Nassau Senior (1831), cited in Black, *Economic Thought and the Irish Question*, p. 92.

56. *Report of the Select Committee on the State of the Poor in Ireland*, pp. 720-2 (ev. of Frederick Page), *HC* (1830), vii.

57. *Royal Commission*, p. 12. As I suggest later, such an argument by the commissioners is indicative of a widespread belief throughout the nineteenth century that the onset of insanity was purely providential, that it owed nothing to the faults of an

individual or his family and antecedents. See below, p. 172n49.

58. K.H. Connell, *The Population of Ireland 1750-1845* (Clarendon Press, Oxford, 1950), p. 201.

59. Cf. Newport's complaint that Waterford is being forced to accommodate the lunatic poor of other counties, *First Report. Minutes of Evidence taken before the Select Committee for the better Regulations of Madhouses in England*, p. 95, *HC* (1816), vi.

60. Under the Act 8 & 9 Vic., c. 126 (1845).

61. MacDonagh, *Ireland*, pp. 34-6 on the weakness of local government in Ireland; *Hansard*, 3rd ser., vol. 76, 619-22 (11 July 1844) for Monteagle (formerly Thomas Spring Rice).

62. *Returns relating to the District Lunatic Asylums in Ireland*, p. 3, *HC* (1839), xliv. See also Appendix, Table A.

63. *22nd Report*, p. 23, *HC* (1873), xxx.

64. *Return of the several Unions in Ireland ... Number of Workhouses ...*, *HC* (1847), xlix; *An Account of the Loans advanced ... for the building of Workhouses ... HC* (1847), lv.

65. See the information on loans prepared for the *Royal Commission on Financial Relations between Great Britain and Ireland*, pp. 462-73, *HC* (1895), xxxvi.

66. Emmet Larkin, 'Economic Growth, Capital Investment, and the Roman Catholic Church', *American Historical Review*, vol. 72 (April 1967), p. 874.

67. See pp. 41-2.

68. *Royal Commission*, p. 5.

69. *Report by the Lords' Select Committee appointed to consider the state of the Lunatic Poor in Ireland*, p. xxv, *HC* (1843), x (hereafter *Lords Committee*).

70. Chief Secretary's Office Registered Papers (hereafter RP) 1845/G8338.

71. RP 1851/3190 (12 December 1845). Cf. Conolly's evidence, *Lords Committee*, ev. 882-3. White had been asked to prepare a report on the possible expansion of the asylum system, following the report of the 1843 Committee, *Report*, pp. 6-7, *HC* (1846), xxii.

72. *Royal Commission*, p. 547.

73. *Report upon the Tables of Death*, p. li, in *Census of Ireland for 1841, HC* (1843), xxiv.

74. RP 1845/G1914.

75. *Report*, p. 18 (1846), xxii.

76. RP 1849/G2869 (for poor law commissioners' survey); *8th Report*, p. 9, *HC* (1875) (II), xvii for the police surveys of 1855 and 1856; the decennial census for 1851 included a comprehensive survey of the insane, within and outside institutions.

77. *Royal Commission*, p. 2; *10th Report*, p. 13, *HC* (1861), xxvii; RP 1887/13281.

78. RP 1849/G3702.

79. RP 1845/G8338.

80. *Report*, p. 59, *HC* (1847), xvii. See also RP 1847/G9236 for the support of the Killarney poor law guardians for these works.

81. RP 1848/G226; RP 1848/G5898.

82. RP 1844/G2392.

83. RP 1845/G8338; RP 1848/G6758 (Fermanagh). *Royal Commission*, p. 544 (Wexford).

84. *4th Report*, p. 16, *HC* (1849), xxiii.

85. *6th Report*, p. 4, *HC* (1852-3), xli.

86. See the preamble (describing administrative arrangements for lunatic asylums) by Thomas Larcom, Under-Secretary at the time, to the volume of correspondence, Larcom Papers, NLI, MS 7775; ibid., Horsman (Chief Secretary) to Larcom, 16 March 1855; and *Select Committee on the Lunatic Asylums (Ireland) (Advances) Bill*, ev. 219-41, *HC* (1854-5), viii.

87. Lunatic Asylums Repayment of Advances (Ireland) Act 18 & 19 Vic., c. 109, s. 6; *Treasury Minutes ... Relating to District Lunatic Asylums (Ireland), HC* (1856), liii.

88. For the controversy and its background, see especially the evidence of Rev. Henry Montgomery, ev. 8034-71, and Francis White, ev. 366-402, *Royal Commission*, and Belfast District Lunatic Asylum, *Minute Books*, HOS 28/1/1/2-3, PRONI.

89. The judgement of the Queen's Bench, in *Rev. John Carroll* v. *Governors and Directors of the Belfast District Lunatic Asylum* (1856) is reprinted in *Royal Commission*, pp. 554-6.

90. Memorandum by Larcom, with note appended, 'Copy to Mr Horsman, 30 April 55', MS 7775/15; Horsman to Larcom, undated, Larcom Papers, NLI, MS 7775/47.

91. Horsman to Carlisle (Lord-Lieutenant), May 1856, MS 7775/53; Fitzgerald (Irish Attorney-General) to Larcom, 21 June 1856, Larcom Papers, NLI, MS 7775/57; *Hansard*, 3rd ser., vol. 142, 1758-65 (20 June 1856): Issac Butt declared that the 'real question was whether a system of central or local government was to be established in Ireland'.

92. Shelley (secretary to the Treasury inquiry) to Larcom, 21 September 1855, Larcom Papers, NLI, MS 7775/26.

93. *Royal Commission*, pp. 1-39.

94. Naas to Larcom, 16 February 1859, Larcom Papers, NLI, MS 7775/93; press cuttings, Larcom Papers, NLI, MS 7776; RP 1859/1782.

95. The board of control was appointed under the 1855 Lunatic Asylum (Advances) (Ireland) Act; for the Privy Council rules see *11th Report*, pp. 55-8, *HC* (1862), xxiii.

96. The Act 30 & 31 Vic., c. 118 (1867) empowered the Lord-Lieutenant to fix the establishment of an asylum and to make an appointment in default of the governors doing so. After further resistance from the Belfast board, the Lord-Lieutenant appointed three chaplains to the asylum in 1869, *19th Report*, p. 11, *HC* (1870), xxxiv.

97. See the advice of T.H. Burke (later Under-Secretary at Dublin Castle), Irish Office, London, to Peel, 8 December 1864, RP 1867/14019; and Nugent's memorandum, 16 February 1866, RP 1867/14019: he reminds government that there was similar opposition in Donegal to a proposed new asylum until he told the people concerned the 'law's powers' in such cases.

98. The schedule of duties of officers and servants in the Richmond lunatic asylum is in *Correspondence regarding Lunatic Asylums in Ireland*, p. 10, *HC* (1828), xxii. Cf. ibid., pp. 23-4, for similar regulations at Armagh. The utopian vision of the asylum under moral management has been well described in Scull, *Museums of Madness*, pp. 102-7.

99. *First Report from Commissioners for Inquiring into the Condition of the Poor in Ireland, Appendix (B)*, pp. 399-400, *HC* (1835), xxxii (Part ii). See *Medical Press and Circular (MPC)*, 16 June 1845 and Williamson, 'Origins of the Irish Mental Hospital Service', pp. 174-7 for the activities of Dr Jacob.

100. Scull, *Museums of Madness*, pp. 148-58; Cf. R.J. Cooter, 'Phrenology and British Alienists, c. 1825-1845', *Medical History*, vol. 20 (1976), pp. 1-21, 135-51.

101. McDowell, *Irish Administration*, p. 173.

102. *Report of the Commissioners appointed to revise the Laws ... Grand Jury Presentments*, Appendix, pp. 98-9, *HC* (1842), xxiv.

103. Ibid., pp. xxxix-xl.

104. 5 & 6 Vic., c. 123, s. 1. It followed the amendment of the English lunacy laws in the same session, 5 & 6 Vic., c. 87. It was Sugden who established the Lord Chancellor's prize for an essay on the treatment of insanity, to be awarded by the College of Physicians in Dublin. T.P.C. Kirkpatrick, *A note on the History of the Care of the Insane in Ireland up to the end of the nineteenth century* (University Press, Dublin, 1931), p. 33.

105. *Lords Committee*, ev. 461, 475, *HC* (1843), x.

106. Ibid., p. xxiii and ev. 466-75 for White's partiality to the position of medical officers in asylums.

107. 8 & 9 Vic., c. 107, s. 23.

108. See Scull, *Museums of Madness*, pp. 152-3 for the opposition in England to a mandatory medical qualification for lunacy inspection. John Nugent (1806-99), MB, Trinity College, Dublin, described in an obituary as 'talented but rash and mischievious', had no previous experience with the insane. His appointment, by a Whig administration, was evidently pure patronage. When White (1787-1859) retired in 1857, following a railway accident in which he was severely injured, patronage again operated to ensure that George Hatchell (?-1890), MD, Glasgow, 1834, household physician to the Lord-Lieutenant, was appointed to replace him. When Nugent and Hatchell retired in 1889 patronage was largely displaced by merit in the appointment of the new inspectors; see below, p. 68. For biographical information on White, Nugent and Hatchell, see Kirkpatrick, *History of the Care of the Insane*, pp. 37-8; *Journal of Mental Science*, vol. 4 (1858), pp. 127-8; ibid., vol. 45 (1899), pp. 431-2.

109. See note 106 above.

110. See 'General Rules for the Government of all the District Lunatic Asylum in Ireland ...', in *Report*, pp. 43-8, *HC* (1844), xxx.

111. *Lords Committee*, ev. 477-9.

112. Ibid., ev. 334.

113. See the questioning of Dr Kidd, Armagh asylum physician, *Select Committee on Medical Charities, Ireland*, ev. 1300-6, *HC* (1843), x.

114. Ibid., ev. 3814-15.

115. *Report*, p. 4, *HC* (1847), xvii.

116. *Dublin Quarterly Journal of Medical Science (DJMS)*, vol. 2 (1846), p. 155; see *MPC*, 28 August 1861, for attribution of authorship to Stewart.

117. *Journal of Psychological Medicine*, vol. 1 (1848), pp. 151-4.

118. *DJMS*, vol. 10 (1850), p. 421.

119. *Royal Commission*, p. 9.

120. See A. Walk and D. Lindsay Walker, 'Gloucester and the beginnings of the RMPA', *Journal of Mental Science (JMS)*, vol. 107 (1961), pp. 603-32 and Scull, *Museums of Madness*, pp. 164-5.

121. *MPC*, 6 August 1851.

122. *JMS*, vol. 3 (1857), pp. 9-11 (English doctor); *DJMS*, vol. 12 (1851), pp. 385-7 (Stewart).

123. *MPC* 11 July 1860; *JMS*, vol. 6 (1860), pp. 522-8. The *Medical Press* had a special interest in the status of the non-resident physicians. John Jacob, the most forceful of them, was a brother of the journal's editor, Arthur Jacob. (I am grateful to Dr J.B. Lyons, library of the Royal College of Surgeons in Ireland, for information on the relationship of the Jacobs.)

124. *JMS*, vol. 7 (1861), pp. 44-9.

125. *MPC*, 18 September 1861—a reply from a defender of Corrigan and the physicians asks 'What test of examination upon mental maladies have these managers undergone?'

126. *JMS*, vol. 7 (1861), p. 280. See RP 1860/11256 for the Maryborough inquiry.

127. *Hansard*, 3rd ser., vol. 164, 1845-50 and vol. 168, 1888. *13th Report*, p. 45, *HC* (1864), xxiii. Blake's arguments and observations are further presented in a pamphlet produced after a tour of Irish and English asylums in the recess of 1861. *Defects in the Moral Treatment of Insanity in the Public Lunatic Asylums of Ireland...* (J.A. Churchill, London, 1862).

128. Cf. *MPC*, 11 September 1861 and 13 November 1861 for support for the non-resident physicians in the *Waterford Mail* and the *Nation*; *JMS*, vol. 8 (1862), p. 351 mentions Privy Council resistance to the new rules.

129. *11th Report*, p. 56, *HC* (1862), xxiii.

2 THE POLITICS OF LUNATIC ASYLUMS, 1867-1914

A corollary of the professionalisation of asylum management was a narrowing of the range of public interest in the problem of lunacy. Inevitably such a tendency would rebound on the doctors' interests, or on those of the institutions they were managing. Thus, discussing asylum dietary in 1886, the superintendent of the Limerick asylum, E.M. Courtenay, admitted that diet was most likely to be raised as a problem in asylum administration in its financial aspect: 'Living as we do in a very poor country, we generally find that all suggestions for improvement are considered under the head of "cost", in the first instance.'[1] For most of the period from the completion of the asylum system in 1870 to the First World War, the financial burden of the institutions was the principal question posed by their existence. The asylum itself had at least a functional legitimacy in Irish society. The public asylums housed some 7,000 inmates in 1870; by 1914 this had trebled to over 21,000, and this was in a society with a declining population. Some anxiety was evident from time to time at the apparently unceasing growth in lunacy which the figures implied. But the increased financial burden was the more significant object of political contention. In 1870 £166,000 was required for the maintenance of the public asylums—this was about one-fifth the amount rated for poor relief in that year. By 1914 £602,000 was levied for lunatics or more than one-half the amount expended on poor relief in that year.[2] Given this tremendous growth it is of little surprise that the fiscal burden constituted the central political question of asylum management before 1914. That is one theme of this chapter.

It is inter-related with another. This same period was dominated by the national question in Ireland. The development of a powerful nationalist politics extended, of course, to a local level as well as to Westminster. In this politics, questions of social policy and administration were largely subordinate to the national question. The emancipation of the nation was taken to be the pre-condition of any necessary social reform; in an extreme form this thinking even seemed to posit Irish independence as a panacea for the country's ills. Consequently asylum administration, in so far as it involved the community, was frequently no more than an arena in which competing political interests could be resolved. This probably exacerbated the

tendency, already evident, to institutional lethargy. The dominance of the national question also explains the relative quiescence in Ireland of the eugenics and social reform movements which so influenced British politics before the war. In Britain the alleged increase of lunacy was seen by many as a symptom of internal decay. The same evidence could be used by John Redmond, in the case of Ireland, as a charge against Britain: 'under your rule', he charged in 1906, 'it has been the survival of the unfittest in Ireland'.[3]

In the absence of these factors—the financial burden, the priority of national self-determination—would Irish asylums have been any different by 1914? The answer, we must suggest, is no. For the third theme of this chapter must be the failure of the lunacy inspectorate. It was from there, principally, that any innovations might have come. But even at its best, the inspectorate's only response to the runaway increase in lunacy was to prescribe more beds and more asylums. At worse, either through their own lethargy, or through the resistance of the ratepayers, the inspectors presided over institutions with serious problems of overcrowding and ill-health. Neither central nor local government before the war could come up with alternatives to the dismal prospect before them. The result, of course, was the survival of institutions of the early nineteenth century well into the succeeding century.

Finance: Ratepayers and the State

From the 1870s lunacy became partly an imperial responsibility; that is, part of the maintenance of the insane in public asylums was reimbursed by the Treasury, the remainder coming from the local rates. It was a Conservative government in 1874 which first took this step but both sides of British politics had previously entertained the idea. Lunacy, as Nassau Senior had argued in the 1830s, was an unpredictable calamity for which neither the individual nor a local community could reasonably be expected to be blamed or responsible. By Edwardian times this view had undergone considerable change: individuals or their ancestors were more readily blamed, though the consequences of this for state policy were complex. But as long as the former view persisted it provided the ideological basis for a policy of state subsidy of asylums. Thus Sir Charles Wood, as Chancellor of the Exchequer in 1851, had proposed to relieve taxation on land by making a payment from the consolidated fund for the relief of lunatics

and idiots in the United Kingdom.[4] As Wood's unsuccessful proposal suggested, such moves owed more to a desire to relieve local taxation than to a well-considered policy of state control of the insane. Before the Edwardian period this latter, wider, view of the question was generally put forward only by the professionals. Joseph Lalor, as president of the Medico-Psychological Association in 1861, argued for the support of the lunatic poor from state funds: many of them, he suggested, were detained like convicts, 'not for their own advantage, but for the protection of society'.[5] In the mid-century decades this was a less cogent consideration for government than the grievance of local taxation and the political uses to which this might be put.

Certainly, by the 1870s both Liberals and Conservatives were seeing the charges for lunatics as in some way an inequitable tax on local communities. In 1869 W.E. Gladstone attempted to incorporate in the Irish Church disestablishment legislation a provision for the application of the surplus arising from the sale of church property to the relief of what he called 'unavoidable calamity and suffering'. A total amount of £311,000 would be made available for the maintenance of the lunatic, idiot and sick poor, removing their charge from the local rates and placing them under the administration of the poor law commissioners.

This proposal, it must be said, did not appear to have arisen from Irish demands. Indeed, like the Irish land legislation of the following year, it had about it some of what Hammond saw as the 'English habit of treating Ireland as a society whose good was to be pursued by English statesmen acting on their own initiative and in their own light'.[6] During the election campaign of 1868 various suggestions had been advanced for the disposal of the church surplus. As Thornley notes, these had ranged from relief of the poor rates through various development projects even to the 'establishment of a tenant proprietary'. But the Gladstone proposal was not enthusiastically received: John Martin, the Nationalist MP, 'considered the devotion of £200,000 a year to the "keeping of poor lunatics" the height of extravagance'.[7] In any case this clause of the Bill was defeated in the Lords where an amendment was passed retaining control of the surplus in the hands of Parliament. Opposition in that House centred on the exclusion of religious purposes from the application of the money. Curiously, in 1869 this seemed to be all that stood in the way of what would, in effect, have been a state take-over of the asylum system.

Had this reform been achieved the administration of asylums and their financial liability would have been substantially altered in the

following fifty years. For the scheme had been originated by the civil servant, John Lambert, with the intention of integrating the asylums in the poor law administration. Though Lambert's proposals were unsuccessful, his report prepared for Gladstone is worth noting for its percipient analysis of the contradictions in Irish local government which failed to be resolved before the turn of the century. County hospitals and district asylums, having been established long before the Irish poor laws, were maintained out of the county cess. This tax was paid by the occupiers (and by them alone) of land of any value. The poor rate, on the other hand, was not assessed on occupiers of land under the value of £4 (about one-quarter of the whole) and for the rest was shared between the tenant and the landlord. Not only was the local taxation system unequal in its burden. In spite of paying most of the cost of hospital and asylum the cesspayers were not represented on the boards of either institution. Instead lunatic asylums were governed (formally at any rate) by nominees of the Lord-Lieutenant, most of them gentry; and the county infirmaries by subscribers who contributed only a fraction of their cost. By bringing these institutions under the poor law, Lambert had hoped to give some say in their management to partly representative bodies and at the same time make their maintenance a 'national' charge.[8] The defeat of these rational reforms ensured the continuing presence of an anachronistic and aggravating local government structure which could become yet another weapon in the nationalist campaign later in the century.

Financial relief, however, was forthcoming before then. While Gladstone's measure would have applied to Ireland alone, the grant in aid of local taxation, introduced by the Conservatives in 1874, applied to both Britain and Ireland. As I have suggested, its introduction was hardly a consequence of Irish demands or pressures. While local taxation had been an important issue in England in the 1874 election, the Irish campaign was dominated by the issues of home rule, denominational education, amnesty for the Fenian prisoners, and land reform. The issue, apparently a peripheral one, which went closest to local taxation in Ireland was the reform of the grand jury system. This was completely unrepresentative of the Catholic tenant majority.[9] So it was popular representation rather than the burden of taxation in itself which was to the forefront of Irish concerns.

The innovation in the financing of lunatic care was a response to pressures within the Conservative Party in England for the alleviation of local taxation. In April 1872, Sir Massey Lopes, the leader of this

lobby, had successfuly moved a resolution to the effect that local taxation should be relieved out of the consolidated fund for charges for justice, police and lunatics. 'Lunacy', he argued in the Commons, 'was a dispensation of Providence, limited to no particular class'. It was a 'national calamity, and should be a national charge and responsibility'.[10] Gladstone's own Irish proposals were cited by Lopes as justification for advancing his motion. As we have already seen, it was a common nineteenth-century view that lunacy, being providential, was a national problem rather than a local one. This view of it, at least, persuaded the Conservative Chancellor of the Exchequer, Sir Stafford Northcote, in his first budget of 1874 to choose the maintenance of lunatics as the means of appeasing the local taxation lobby. If local taxation was inequitable, the Chancellor argued, social measures to reinforce the 'condition of the people' would meet local resistance. To smooth the way for the implementation of what he called 'our social policy' the Treasury would grant a fixed rate of four shillings per head per week for the maintenance of lunatics in public asylums in Britain and Ireland.[11] What effect did this grant have on the lunatic asylums in Ireland?

From the beginning there was an ambiguity about the purpose and a confusion about the mode of administering the grant. To the inspectors of lunatics the government's measure was not so much a relief to local taxation as a contribution to the improvement of asylums. This was a misreading of the spirit of the grant which Northcote had implied would enable local authorities to pursue properly local objects: town improvements, housing and so on. The inspectors saw it instead as in part their property, an instrument of government which could be used to expand asylum accommodation and improve facilities. Since the government now paid 'fully two-fifths of [the lunatics'] maintenance' they suggested that central intervention was warranted in 1876 in forcing the Derry and Armagh boards to undertake new works.[12] Instead of a contraction in expenditure they wanted a more liberal administration on the part of local authorities. Yet, given the grant's purpose of reducing local taxation, it was hardly surprising that many asylum boards did what they could to throw as much of the burden as possible onto the Treasury.

In fact the administration of the grant ensured that the Treasury, at least until 1890, bore an increasing portion of the total cost of Irish asylums. While the Chancellor had implied that the four shillings per week was a fixed rate, the Treasury had 'presumed' in 1874 that the government's contribution would not exceed half the net cost of the

lunatic's maintenance, that is in some cases it would be below four shillings.[13] This was not the understanding originally taken by Dublin Castle.[14] And in practice the full amount of four shillings, regardless of the level of total expenditure, was usually granted. Consequently, at a time of growing numbers of inmates and increased total cost, the Treasury contribution climbed throughout the 1880s to constitute over 50 per cent of asylum maintenance by 1886-8.[15] In some asylums, like that at Omagh, the Treasury was paying as much as 65 per cent by the late 1880s: the Omagh governors, reported the inspectors of lunatics in 1890, had received in the previous five years about £6,000 more than the figure to which the Treasury conditions had strictly entitled them. By this time there were two new inspectors, eager to expand accommodation and improve conditions in the many overcrowded asylums. It was they who prompted a tightening-up of administration to ensure that local boards did not receive more than their due share. The grant, administered faultily as it had been, was alleged by the inspectors to have curtailed the comforts of inmates and frustrated the 'beneficent intention of the Government ... to improve the condition of the insane'.[16]

In fact, of course, there had been no such 'beneficent intention'. The measure, though a substantial innovation in the financing of a public service, had been purely pragmatic. It was an administrative device whose beneficent intention was to relieve the ratepayer rather than improve the condition of the lunatic. It was not founded on any substantial consideration of what responsibility central government had for the insane or why it should assume such a responsibility. Consequently, while inspectors attempted rather fruitlessly to use some moral blackmail on intransigent local authorities, the lunatic asylums remained much the same as they had been before 1874, if a little more crowded. Finally it was not even clear that the declining proportion of local contributions to maintenance was the result of a conscious choice by parsimonious asylum boards and grand juries. The main reason for the apparent reduction in the local share in the 1880s was probably the agricultural depression. Agricultural prices dropped by the order of 20-30 per cent between the mid 1870s and late 1880s.[17] Since 'provisions' were the major component (over 40 per cent)[18] of asylum costs, a dramatic decline in agricultural prices reduced the average cost of keeping a lunatic in an asylum. With this reduction asylums which had a tradition of cheap maintenance costs dropped below the eight shillings a week average which formally entitled them to the maximum Treasury aid. This, rather than

malfeasance on the part of asylum governors, explained the growing imbalance of local and Treasury contributions. With the re-establishment of Treasury control over the estimation of the grant after 1890 the Treasury share of asylum finance dropped back to the original level of 40 per cent by 1898.

In spite of the substantial role of central government in the financing of lunatic care after 1874 there was little change in the nature of asylum administration. In fact the asylums in Ireland were in a phase of stagnation. An aged and complacent inspectorate, the decline of which we will examine later, did not help matters. The one sign of change stemmed principally from the rise of home rule politics though there was also a surviving element of the struggles of the 1850s between local and central authority. In the 1880s and 1890s governments were constantly presented with a demand for ratepayers' control of asylum administration. It was a demand which derived both from a nationalist desire for self-determination and from a concern with increasing costs, even in spite of the Treasury contributions.

In the 1850s the call for local control had been one on behalf of the rural landed gentry who dominated the grand juries and thereby the asylum boards. By the 1870s grievances about local government focused on the lack of representation of taxpayers on these bodies. A deputation to the Lord-Lieutenant (Spencer) and Chief Secretary (Hartington) in January 1873 urged the necessity of such representation. The deputation represented mainly urban interests: the city corporations did not even have the representation on asylum boards which county grand jurys usually had. Sir Dominic Corrigan, the Dublin MP and former medical professor, strongly attacked the administration of asylums, the escalating costs and the lack of any means by which ratepayers could exert control over these costs. The financial question was of central concern to the deputation. Representation was seen as a way of controlling costs, an illusion which only the achievement of representation would dispel.[19] Similarly a number of witnesses before the 1868 select committee on Irish grand jury presentments had seen representation of cesspayers on asylum boards as a means of achieving economies. No charge on the county cess had increased as enormously in the previous twenty years as that for lunatics.[20]

In spite of the Liberal administration's sympathy with the ratepayers' grievance nothing was done before the 1874 election which returned the Conservatives to power. The 1874 grant both advanced and weakened the ratepayers' cause—the rates were relieved but the sizeable central contribution now limited the case for locally elected

asylum boards. Nevertheless the claims for representation continued and sometimes local concessions were won. The Limerick asylum board was forced in 1874 to allow a committee of Limerick corporation to examine the accounts and inspect the asylum.[21] Much effort was expended later in the decade in investigating the anomalies of Irish local government and taxation. Yet the only legislative attempt to reform the grand jury laws, in 1878, lapsed in the face of opposition from home rulers who found it too limited in scope.[22]

In the absence of thorough-going reform, governments in the 1880s and 1890s tended to concede at least symbolic representation where local interests were felt to be under-represented. Early in the 1880s a Liberal Chief Secretary, W.E. Forster, allowed the Cork corporation to suggest three members for appointment to the asylum board. A request by Limerick for similar treatment was turned down by Forster because, he claimed, the city already had adequate representation among the governors.[23] In any case the Liberal administration made no attempt to grapple with local government reform. It was left to the Conservatives, with their penchant for domestic reforms, to take the steam out of home rule and to restructure the asylum boards.

Already in January 1887 Dublin Castle had begun to clear the dead wood from the lists of governors, the majority of whom—gentry, bishops and magistrates—never attended board meetings. Over one hundred governors who had not attended one board meeting in the previous three years were expunged from the boards.[24] Still this stopped short of the desire of urban interests. Late in 1887 the Dublin corporation decided to postpone the presentment of asylum maintenance charges until they received satisfaction in their demands for representation.[25] Desiring some change itself, the government responded in November 1888 with a reconstitution of asylum boards: half the members would be nominated by the government, the rest selected by the Viceroy from nominations of the county grand jurys and city corporations, in proportion to their respective financial contributions. This measure of proportionate representation was what the Dublin authorities in particular had wanted. Having a large population of immigrant workers and the poor, the city supported the greater number of the inmates of the largest asylum in Ireland, yet up till 1888 had no formal say in asylum management.[26]

By this stage, however, the struggle over the structure of asylum boards was not only concerned with taxation and representation. As the attitude of the Cork corporation and the government's response demonstrates, the asylum boards, like the poor law boards before

them, were becoming the focus of nationalist infiltration. Invited by the government to send a list of nominations for its four seats on the asylum board, the Cork councillors sent only four names. The four, reported the resident magistrate confidentially to Dublin, were 'advanced Nationalists'. The Lord-Lieutenant refused to appoint them, selecting his own representatives from among the compliant members of the council. Consequently the council refused to present for the asylum in September 1889 and the government was forced to undertake protracted legal action to obtain the money.[27] The Conservatives had breached the old order but clearly wanted to retain the government's right to oversee local government and control the incursions of nationalism. Nevertheless a Liberal Chief Secretary, John Morley, was soon to use his rights of appointment to effectively challenge ascendancy dominance of local administration.

Prepared to leave the future reform of local government to the Irish themselves under home rule, the Liberal government undertook in the meantime to 'democratise' some Irish institutions by redressing the Protestant dominance of the magistracy and of asylum boards.[28] The autocratic removal of Protestant governors and their replacement by Catholics horrified some Unionists, one of whom thought some of the new 'untried men' were of 'the lowest character'.[29] But Morley was on safe ground, being able to refer to the Conservative government's unsuccessful Local Government Bill of 1892 which would have made the asylum boards dependent on popular elections.[30] His proposal did not invite this danger.

The breach which had been made in the old order was soon to be widened by legislation. Home rule had failed. So had the first attempt by the Conservatives to reform local government—their half-hearted Bill of 1892, which was so hedged with qualifications to protect the interests of the Unionists in local politics. But after the Unionists returned to office in 1895 a more honest and conciliatory measure was prepared. Local government reform was, of course, part of the 'constructive' Unionist platform; it had been in the offing since 1886 and was, in essence, the Unionist substitute for home rule. The general story has been told elsewhere so it will be more useful here to examine how exactly it affected one institution of local politics, the asylum board.[31]

The major effect of the reform was the transfer of the non-judicial duties of grand juries to popularly-elected county councils.[32] The councils were required, under section 9, to provide and maintain sufficient accommodation for the insane poor, as set out in the various

Lunacy Acts. Some vestiges of the old order were left—the Lord-Lieutenant might order the council to remedy any deficiencies in the council's provision for the lunatic poor. But otherwise central powers were truncated—the board of control which had been responsible for the planning and construction of the asylums since the 1820s was abolished; asylum rules were now to be drafted by each asylum individually, although the appproval of the Lord-Lieutenant was required. Most important of all, the county councils might appoint and remove all officers of the asylum (including the medical superintendent), and regulate the expenditure; the powers of the Lord-Lieutenant and the inspectors of lunatics in these matters were to cease. Hence the inspectors' role was considerably modified, away from administration and control towards an affirmation of truly inspectorial duties. The boards of governors were to be replaced by committees appointed by the council, mostly from its own members; where two or more councils comprised one district the finances and the representation on the committee were to be in proportion to the number of inmates from each county. In line with this large-scale transfer of responsibility to local authorities the government also strictly delimited its own financial commitment for the future. The various grants-in-aid of the rates were to cease. Instead the Treasury would pay a sum equal to the proceeds of the previous year's local taxation (that is mainly from liquor licences) together with a fixed grant of £79,000, into a local taxation (Ireland) account. From this the Lord-Lieutenant would order payments to local authorities on account of the lunatic poor at the rate of four shillings per week or half the average cost of maintenance, whichever was the less. While section 9 had clearly devolved power from Dublin to the local authorities, section 58 meant that the Lord-Lieutenant (and thereby the inspectors of lunatics) retained some control—the payments would be made on condition that the county councils had fulfilled their duties to the lunatic poor. The extent to which a government might be prepared to use this condition was, of course, a subtle matter. It was probably of very limited use in the context of Irish politics after 1898. Nationalist-dominated councils were to become even more resistant to Dublin Castle directives until in the end there was a wholesale subversion of British administration. Arthur Balfour had reason to fear that the nationalists would use local government reform as 'a ladder by which to climb to Home Rule, and possibly through Home Rule to separation'.[33]

There was no doubt that the reform was a thorough one. Politically,

it was long overdue. Financially, its consequences for lunatic asylums were not clearly seen in 1898 but some were aware of them. A conference of asylum governors in Dublin in April was anxious about the possible future abatement of the lunatic grant. Given the continuing increase of asylum inmates, the relatively fixed fund for their maintenance might soon be exhausted.[34] Of the Irish parliamentarians, only John Dillon questioned the wisdom of the financial clauses, though he thought the Bill itself 'a great and liberal measure'.[35] His warning that the fund would soon be exhausted proved true within ten years. What the government did in 1898 (and had done in England and Scotland ten years before) was to set a limit on its own contribution to the care of lunatics and hand back the burden as well as the responsibility to the local authorities.

The Decline of the Inspectorate

The predominance of questions of finance and local control over asylums in the decades after 1870 was aided and abetted by a decline in the authority of the inspectorate. Aside from a brief period in the 1890s this arm of central control demonstrated an inability to pursue anything more than a routine administrative role during this period. In part this was a problem of personnel: in the 1880s the two inspectors were aged, even invalid, and had little energy to carry out their duties efficiently. Yet even with new inspectors appointed in 1890 there was little imagination shown in administration or policy. And after the local government reform of 1898 the authority of Dublin Castle was limited in law and practice. Throughout the pre-war period it was clear to the inspectors that no longer could they expect local authorities to heed their admonitions or advice.

The first inspector, Francis White, had been the dominant figure in the consolidation of the asylum system in the 1840s. However, with White's retirement in 1857 it was the second inspector, John Nugent, whose style quickly came to dominate the image of the inspectorate. A vigorous advocate of his department's interests (but with a narrow vision of what those interests were) he was not averse to intervening behind the scenes at Westminster to achieve his ends. In 1859 he lobbied against Lord Naas' Irish Lunacy Bill which limited Dublin Castle's control over the asylum system.[36] With church disestablishment imminent, he wrote at least four times in 1869 to Chichester Fortescue, the Chief Secretary, for the allocation of the church

surplus to public asylums. This, he argued, should be accompanied by a reversion to the government of the power of appointments to asylum positions.[37] Such a move would, of course, have served to greatly increase the standing and power of his own office. As with George Hatchell, his fellow inspector who succeeded Francis White, it is doubtful whether Nugent had any experience of lunatic asylums prior to his appointment. During more than forty years of office he failed to show that his conception of his role went any further than a rather mundane administration of institutions. At the same time the inspectorate's faults were compounded by a confused division of responsibilities between the various parties responsible for asylums and by the indecision of the Irish government in determining who should control the asylums.

The division of responsibilities for the care of lunatics was the crux of many a dispute between the three groups concerned—namely the inspectors of lunatics, the boards of governors and the medical superintendents. As Nugent pointed out on the eve of his retirement, the title of 'Inspectors' was somewhat misleading since it implied that their duties were 'essentially inspectorial'.[38] Yet their duties were also administrative, and to a very large degree this latter role became the more important one. Being administratively responsible for the institutions they were supposed to inspect imposed a conflict of interest. From 1860, the inspectors were members of the board of control, the body whose duty was the planning and construction of district asylums. As well they had been *ex officio* members of all asylum boards from 1853 until 1861.[39] Criticism of the Irish asylum system, of the buildings themselves, or of the conditions of those confined in them, could thus implicitly become criticism of the efficiency and competence of the 'inspectorial administration'. This was not the limit of the inspectors' conflicts of interest. Both Nugent and Hatchell (and indeed all inspectors between 1845 and 1921) were medical men. Moreover, Nugent was a member, though not an active one, of the Medico-Psychological Association, the professional organisation of asylum doctors. His sympathies were thus very much with that side of the medical profession—a fact which partly explains the animus of some of the attacks on him by the *Medical Press and Circular*, a journal which was much attached to private practice and the consultancy system. Finally, the multilateral commitments existed even at a personal level—the inspector George Hatchell was father of two of the twenty-two district asylum superintendents in the later 1880s.[40]

Clearly the possibilities of impartial inquiry into the conditions of asylums generally and into cases of ill-treatment more specifically must have been limited by the inspectors' ubiquitous presence in the various levels of asylum administration. This situation not only led to cover-ups and apologetics but also to acrimonious, lengthy and distracting disputes between inspectors and boards of governors, between governors and superintendents and even between inspectors and superintendents. If only because of its implications for the standard of treatment and conditions in asylums, this disintegration of the inspectorate in the 1870s and 1880s bears investigation.

The nature of these conflicts was evident in the aftermath of the Danford case at Limerick asylum. On 2 December 1871, James Danford died after being given a plunge-bath by an attendant whom he had struck. The bath had been authorised by the superintendent, Dr Fitzgerald. After Danford's death Fitzgerald had entered it in the daily statement book but later partly obliterated the circumstances from the book, and did not report the death to the coroner (unlike English practice, or at least prescription, the reporting of asylum deaths to a coroner was not mandatory at the time in Ireland).[41] In four inspections of the asylum after this date Nugent appeared to absolve the superintendent from responsibility and suggested the prosecution of the attendant. But, in addition, he criticised the governors for failing to draw his attention to the manner of Danford's death, and their failure to make regular inspections of the asylum. This was too much for the board which, in the following months, agitated for an inquiry into Nugent's conduct of the case, his own alleged failings in the matter of inspection and his whitewashing of the superintendent. When the attendant was subsequently prosecuted but acquitted Dr Fitzgerald resigned, though evidently to Nugent's regret. This was not the end of the dispute which raged on into the early months of 1874. The board charged that everything in the administration of asylums went to increase the authority of the inspectors; in particular amendments to the Privy Council rules and regulations in recent years had subverted the governors' authority, transferring it to the inspectors and the medical superintendent.[42] The case revealed the fissures in the confusing administrative structure. The governors could hide their own failings in the management of the asylum in claiming that proper inspection was the inspectors' responsibility; the superintendent whose actions, notably in concealing the circumstances of Danford's death,[43] were inexcusable was protected (at least initially) by the inspector's professional sympathy; the inspectorate itself was compro-

mised by the provocative Nugent who one moment was an administrator, the next an inspector. Perhaps it was because of the trouble created for the government in this case that a rumour circulated about this time that the Irish lunacy service would be placed under the local government board. The *Medical Press* welcomed the likely fall of 'Nugent's dictatorship'.[44]

At this time the inspectors faced attacks not only from below but also from above. T.H. Burke, the Under-Secretary who had to defend Nugent against the Limerick board in 1873, was himself clearly dissatisfied with the competence of the lunatic asylums office. The inspectors' parliamentary reports were frequently presented very late; after an extended delay in the 1874 report Burke asked Herbert Murray, a Treasury official, to inquire into the office. While a previous such inquiry had evidently been favourable, Murray's report in 1876 criticised the efficiency of the office, recommended the abolition of the chief clerkship (vacated the previous year by William Corbet, later a Parnellite MP for Wicklow) and advocated, in effect, a truncation of the annual report. Murray found that the report of 1873 had been written by the chief clerk and not by the inspectors. In defence the inspectors replied that Mr Murray seemed to 'favour a restricted Estimate of the requirements of a Lunacy Department of Ireland' (that is no chief clerkship in the office). But Burke directed them to change the style of the annual reports and to prepare them personally.[45] Throughout the decade Burke was led to question the inspectors' efficiency and mode of carrying out their duties. In the wake of the Danford case, Burke inquired, on behalf of the Lord-Lieutenant, into the inspection of lunatics in *poorhouses*. This duty was clearly required of the inspectors by statute but they could only lamely reply that it would be impossible to visit every workhouse which kept lunatics.[46] Later this apology became a defence of their failure to notice abuses in asylums.[47] It was obviously an impossible task to examine all the inmates of the asylum so attention tended to wander in the direction of administration.

If Nugent erred in one way in not doing what he was supposed to do, he equally was inclined to provoke by intervening arbitrarily *ultra vires*. The College of Physicians was incensed by his behaviour on one such occasion when he used his position to overrule the refusal by a private asylum doctor to allow a visitor to see a patient in his asylum. Burke, having communicated with the Solicitor-General and the English commissioners in lunacy, rebuked Nugent for this interference beyond his statutory powers.[48] One might sympathise with this action

in favour of the patient (or it might have been the visitor) but for Nugent's disregard of the rights of the patient on other occasions. Although the government law adviser thought it a 'very reasonable thing to show a man, when he is sane, the documents by virtue of which he has been detained in a lunatic asylum', the inspectors refused in 1878 to release committal documents to a discharged inmate of the Richmond asylum.[49]

Widespread dissatisfaction with the inspectorate in the 1870s was followed by a wholesale lack of confidence in the personnel and the system in the 1880s. For much of the decade one inspector, George Hatchell, was ill and unable to perform his duties.[50] Nugent, who turned 80 in 1886, was therefore left with the bulk of the duties. His poor personal relations with individuals in the asylum service continued. In 1883 the Assistant Under-Secretary had to conduct a full-scale inquiry into the animosity between Nugent and Lalor, the medical superintendent of the Richmond asylum, which was said by the asylum board to be interfering with the 'proper management and discipline of the Establishment'.[51] After this episode Dublin Castle lost all confidence in the inspectorate. Indeed a government Bill in 1883 included a clause to bring the lunatic asylums under the control of the medical inspectors of the local government board.[52] Other provisions in the Bill led to its withdrawal but the incompetence of the inspectorate forced the government and the Castle to look elsewhere for advice on the asylums. The quality of the inspectors' reports had deteriorated and their memoranda for the Under-Secretary were scarcely noticed. 'The Inspectors' remarks are of no value whatever for the purpose in view', commented an irritated Irish Office clerk trying to prepare an answer to a parliamentary question in 1887.[53]

In this situation the government resorted instead to the use of other public officials. Arthur Mitchell, a Scottish lunacy commissioner, was asked by Dublin Castle to inquire into at least three separate Irish lunacy matters in 1885: the need for a new asylum in the Cavan and Monaghan district, the state of the lunatic wards in the south Dublin workhouse, and the large number of escapes from the Dundrum criminal asylum.[54] All were matters ordinarily the responsibility of the lunacy inspectors. On the last inquiry Mitchell was joined by R.W.A. Holmes, the Treasury remembrancer for Ireland. In January 1889 Arthur Balfour, the Chief Secretary, appointed these two men with Dr F.X.F. MacCabe, a medical inspector with the local government board, to inquire into the state of Irish lunacy administration.[55] The inquiry had finally been prompted by the demand of the

Donegal board for the abolition of the lunatic asylums' office which the board considered no longer adequate to its duties. Even following the receipt of this complaint and the appointment of the committee of inquiry the Donegal board failed to get satisfaction from the inspectorate. The board's request of 8 January 1889 for the inspectors to investigate three cases of solitary confinement, one of which had resulted in a death, was not followed up by Nugent until early April.[56] Hatchell retired in February 1889, Nugent later the same year, after a marathon tenure of 43 years.

Considering the circumstances under which the Mitchell committee had been appointed and the strong pressures within the bureaucracy to transfer the inspectorate to the local government board the report's recommendations were a surprise.[57] In fact the main recommendation was exactly what Nugent had always argued for: the committee thought that it would be best to establish a lunacy board, as in England and Scotland. Lunacy administration, so the report argued, was too large and important a business to be added to a board already burdened with other responsibilities. In default of this change, which would require legislation, the board of control was to be revived with full powers to regulate asylums (previously it had largely been lunacy administration (the essentials of which were forty years also include a number of persons 'of good business habits, who are not officials but have leisure' and an interest in the 'amelioration of the insane'. No doubt this would conciliate the ratepayers by controlling bureaucratic extravagance. Asked whether it was necessary to have more than one inspector the committee reported that *at least* two were required. The report was strongly stamped with the model of Scottish lunacy administration (the essentials of which were forty years younger than the Irish system), so much so that a glossary of terms explaining the Scottish system was included.

Given the government's reluctance to establish a separate lunacy board, the Mitchell committee's report did not initiate a new era in asylum administration. Instead its strong opposition to the incorporation of asylums in the local government board ensured the survival of the inspectorate. In 1890 Dublin Castle chose two energetic and well-qualified medical men to succeed Nugent and Hatchell. Unlike the appointments made fifty years earlier these were undoubtedly made chiefly on the basis of merit. Both men had distinguished student careers at Trinity College. After some years private practice in Boyle, Co. Roscommon, George Plunkett O'Farrell had been appointed a medical inspector to the local government board in 1885; in 1888 he

was appointed medical member of the general prisons board and inspector of reformatory and industrial schools. Although he had not worked in an asylum he had experience of investigating the condition of lunatics in workhouses. E. Maziere Courtenay had taken first place in the Trinity MB in 1871. He was then assistant medical officer in the Derby county asylum before succeeding Dr Fitzgerald (of Danford case notoriety) as superintendent of the Limerick asylum in 1874. He was an active member of the Medico-Psychological Association, having been primarily responsible for establishing its Irish branch. His appointment ('entirely due to his name and reputation as an authority in lunacy', according to an official minute) was therefore particularly welcome to the aspiring professionals of that association and especially to the Irish asylum medical officers.[58] The *Journal of Mental Science* hoped these appointments would redeem the character of Irish asylums and raise the level of the specialty, previously neglected in Ireland.[59]

The new inspectors threw themselves into their work with a sense of mission, discovering abuses, negligence and degeneration of the system wherever they went. In July 1890 they reported to the Under-Secretary on the steps taken in connection with lunacy administration since the appointment of the Mitchell committee. They had adopted the procedure of the English lunacy commissioners, visiting each asylum together and then forwarding inspection reports to the asylum board, to the government and to the board of control; they pursued the same routine in inspecting private asylums and had recommended the revocation of one licence. They proposed appointing a small committee into the administration of the Dundrum asylum. And they were proposing that the revived and strengthened board of control (now with four non-official members, in addition to the chairman of the board of works and themselves) should concern itself with the regulation and management of the asylum as well as asylum construction and land purchase.[60] This view of the future, in essence an attempt to create a lunacy board on the English and Scottish model, was rather too ambitious: the new chairman of the board of control, Justice Holmes argued that the statutory powers (under the 1821 Act) did not enable the board to interfere in the regulation and management of asylums.[61]

In their early years the new inspectors found much to occupy them in calculating the deteriorated state of asylum care. In July 1890 the *Medical Press* applauded their energy—they had just recently thrown 'bomb-shells' among the Armagh and Omagh guardians by their

reports on the state of the lunatic wards in workhouses. The new inspectors evidently would not be content with 'the stereotyped eulogistic report which has been the unchanging fashion of past years'.[62] Apart from the endemic overcrowding (the consequence of increasing admission rates in the previous decade) the first annual report by O'Farrell and Courtenay criticised the inadequate facilities for employment of the inmates and the lack of space in Irish asylums. These deficiencies, they alleged, led to the unwarranted use of mechanical restraint in some asylums and to the confinement of refractory patients in depressing, closed-in courtyards.[63] Their most vigorous attack, however, was reserved for the state of workhouse accommodation for lunatics. In the workhouses, there was little control of the quality of care; pauper inmates were sometimes in charge of the lunatics and able to use mechanical restraint to control them.[64] In the South Dublin union workhouse the shower-bath, 'a relic of the barbarous treatment of the insane', had been introduced and was evidently used as a punishment by the resident physician.[65]

By sending a report on each inspection to the asylum board the inspectors, in effect, made public the state of each institution and thereby encouraged improvements—the Cork asylum board was so stung by one report that it refused to release it to the press; yet before long new buildings for over four hundred patients were being planned.[66] In their second report the inspectors dwelt at length on the need for expanded facilities. They were doubtful of the long-term effectiveness of auxiliary asylums or converted workhouses, the economical alternatives. Instead, they argued, a greater 'liberality' of expenditure was part of a real economy in the care of the insane: the 1875 *Lancet* commission on asylums was cited to reinforce their case. To encourage the governors they supported the move for an extension of the period of repayment of Treasury loans from fourteen to twenty years.[67] They were soon arguing for a further easing of the loan conditions to enable repayment over thirty-five or even fifty years, similar to loans for labourers' dwellings.[68] By the middle of the decade these long-term loans were being granted for asylum construction. Hence the inspectors were able to use the promise of cheaper finance to persuade local authorities to engage in some massive new works.[69] Protests by Derry ratepayers against the new county asylum were met by the inspectors with the reply that the repayments for the £100,000 asylum would be extended over fifty years.[70]

The rate of asylum expansion during these years was astonishing. Every annual report during the 1890s included an impressive list of

asylums being built anew, expanded or substantially renovated. In 1894, for instance, new asylums were being planned for Holywell (to serve Co. Antrim), Belfast, Derry and Portrane (as a second asylum for the Richmond district); detached hospital blocks were being constructed at Armagh (150 beds) and Ballinasloe (200 beds); and substantial new blocks were being planned or built at Clonmel, Carlow, Maryborough and Waterford. At Cork, in spite of the recent completion of extra accommodation for 400 inmates, the inspectors warned that further buildings would be required or alternative accommodation sought.[71]

In spite of their enthusiasm for renovation, the inspectors' vision of lunacy care was essentially narrow and inflexible. Inevitably, as the addition of more and more asylum beds failed to keep pace with the demand on facilities, local authorities became restive, even resistant to the inspectors' programme of expansion. After 1898 asylum committees appointed by popularly-elected local government bodies had the power to ignore the directives of Dublin Castle. In the meantime unhappiness with the vicious circle of expansion and over-crowding brought to the surface some alternative policies for the care of the insane. The inspectors' opposition to anything less than, or even different from, the relatively expensive standards of district asylum accommodation can only have contributed to the decline in authority of their office.

The most common alternative proposed by asylum boards was the maintenance of the so-called chronic and incurable classes in workhouses or in disused workhouses converted into auxiliary asylums. Legislation of 1875 had, in fact, empowered asylum authorities to contract with workhouses for the care of harmless lunatics. Only in isolated cases (the Ballymena workhouse housed over 100 patients from Belfast asylum in the 1890s) was the legislation used. Asylum authorities preferred to use another section of the same Act to discharge the harmless, leaving the workhouse to care for them as destitute.[72] Another economical mode of institution-alisation was the auxiliary asylum: a workhouse or gaol converted into a low-grade, custodial lunatic asylum. The Mitchell committee had given its qualified support to this alternative. Yet whenever specific proposals were made the inspectors were vehement in their opposition. While Mitchell had questioned the feasibility of conversion in particular instances (the Gortin workhouse in Co. Tyrone had been suggested) the inspectors considered workhouse buildings in general as unsuitable and the amount of land available insufficient for the

'treatment and employment of the Insane'.[73] Even when local government reform in 1898 provided for the establishment of auxiliary asylums the government offered only half the grant *per capita* paid for inmates in district asylums (that is a maximum of two shillings instead of four). This, together with the inspectors' determination that the care of lunatics be at a level considerably above that offered in the workhouse, meant that an 'economical' asylum was an impossibility. The inspectors' policy was sound enough in reason but local authorities saw in it only obstruction and financial burden.

The inspectors' suspicion of innovation was also evident in their reaction to the possibility of 'boarding-out'. This practice, whereby some asylum inmates were boarded out with families, was extensively practised in Scotland. At the prompting of Conolly Norman, medical superintendent of the Richmond asylum, its extension to Ireland was urged by the Richmond board after 1898. In spite of the arguments in its favour (its humanity, its economy) the inspectors were less than enthusiastic. It would be difficult to find suitable, cleanly houses and avoid the temptation to make a profit at the patient's expense; property values might be threatened; the public outcry which would follow any abuses of the system, assaults or outrages committed by or against the patients, would be greater in Ireland than in Scotland; the danger of some being committed to the asylum with the intent of having them sent home again as state-supported boarders; the lack of respect for the law in Ireland which might lead to disregard of regulations. Although they were prepared to see a limited scheme (under their own control, not under the asylum committees) introduced, their minute cast doubt over the whole idea. Consequently, halting attempts to draw up an appropriate Bill in 1901 and 1904 failed.[74]

A state-controlled and financed asylum system was the one demand of local authorities which the inspectors were unlikely to oppose. From 1880 local opinion occasionally favoured this step, citing the 1877 state take-over of prisons as a precedent.[75] The Co. Derry grand jury in 1880 saw the Treasury grant from 1874, the Gladstone proposals of 1869 and the transfer of the prisons to the Exchequer as all having established the 'principle' of the liability of all property to maintain the insane poor.[76] The release of the report of the financial relations commission in 1895, concluding that Ireland was over-taxed, brought numerous memorials to government from grand juries and asylum boards, requesting that the entire maintenance of the insane poor be paid out of imperial funds. The calls continued into 1897 and 1898.[77] However, as we have seen, the government had no

intention of committing itself financially to the maintenance of all lunatics in Ireland. Unlike the prison population which was declining in the later nineteenth century, the asylum population increase showed no sign of abating. In 1898 the government was careful to limit its financial liability in the future. The consequence was to be a growing burden for local taxation and a burgeoning conflict between asylum committees and Dublin Castle.

Social Policy and the Politics of Nationalism

Fundamental differences between the domestic concerns of Irish and British politics became ever more obvious in the early years of the new century. In Britain the need for social reform to preserve the nation's imperial position became a major preoccupation. In Ireland the politics of nationalism predominated over the voice of those who sought domestic regeneration within the prevailing framework of the Union with Britain. In Britain the new visibility of the 'degenerate' poor, magnified by the setbacks of the Boer War, was the signal for an obsession with the rejuvenation of British society. This led to a questioning of the institutions created by the nineteenth-century state, to a concern with poor law reform, health insurance and care, unemployment and its remedies. In Ireland on the other hand, the condition of the people—signified by high emigration, declining marriage, or even increasing lunacy—was taken to be symptomatic of the decay of the nation. Conveniently, Irish nationalist rhetoric could blame this on British rule in Ireland rather than on the Irish social structures and institutions. 'Under your rule', John Redmond charged in the Commons in 1906, 'it has been the survival of the unfittest in Ireland'.[78] He was referring to the alleged increase in lunacy. For this reason, and by this logic, the Irish priority was self-determination, the necessary prelude to any social reform.

Hence it is not surprising that the lunatic asylum system and its administration stagnated in Ireland during these years. A major change in the balance of power in the system had been made in 1898 —the politics of nationalism in all its ramifications also dominated the public asylums. The Local Government Act of 1898, comments F.S.L. Lyons,

had provided an outlet for the initiative and energies of a great number of nationalists, an outlet all the more highly prized since self-government on the national scale was still denied.[79]

What this meant when applied to an asylum committee was an unwillingness to spend more money on buildings, nationalist patronage in the appointment of staff, the politicisation of committee meetings, in short, the beginnings of that process of subversion which culminated in the breakdown of British administration in Ireland after the war. In this concluding section we will briefly examine the reasons for the stagnation of the lunacy question in Ireland after 1898.

The immediate effect of the reform of local government was to 'nationalise' asylum management. Protestant-dominated asylum boards overnight became Catholic-dominated committees of management. Not all was smooth going in this transition: the Belfast Catholic Association protested in June 1899 that the Belfast City Council had nominated only three Catholics, as opposed to eighteen Protestants, to the Belfast asylum committee.[80] But in most areas of Ireland the new arrangements made Catholic and nationalist domination of the asylum committees a foregone conclusion. The implications of this fact no doubt varied from area to area. But some committees were intent on leaving their imprint on the asylum staff. In 1904 the junior assistant medical officer at Ballinasloe, Dr Kirwan, was appointed superintendent over the head of his senior, Dr Mills, a Protestant. Since the Lord-Lieutenant's concurrence in the appointment was necessary, the government inquired why Mills had been passed over. But the new limits on the government's power were evident in its ineffectual protest. The committee denied the right of anyone to demand a reason for its vote. The government lamely replied that it did have the right and that the appointment of a junior officer was 'of doubtful expedience'; but since it was not prohibited by the Act, the Lord-Lieutenant would not withhold his agreement. Conservative newspapers in Belfast and Dublin were agitated about the appointment —the *Belfast Newsletter* claimed that Dr Kirwan was described as the 'mainstay, the support and the corner-stone of the St Grella's Branch' of the Gaelic League. In a later interview with an *Irish Times* reporter Kirwan discussed his nationalist sympathies and some changes he had made in the asylum since his appointment. He and the committee had decided to replace the buttons on the attendants' uniforms, which bore an insignia of the crown, with ones bearing the harp and shamrock. He had also ordered new stationery embossed 'On the People's Service', although he only used these locally and still used the old 'OHMS' envelopes in correspondence with Dublin Castle.[81] After this episode the nationalist sympathies of the Ballinasloe committee can have been in no doubt; perhaps it was useful for Mr P.

Carey, applying for a position as asylum attendant, to have the Aughrim Hurling Club recommend him to the committee in 1907. Other committees, particularly in the west, were subject to similar pressures. Early in 1901 the Calry branch of the United Irish League wrote to the Sligo asylum committee protesting against the appointment of Miss Boylan as an attendant as she was the daughter of 'an enemy to the people's organization', a man who was a 'bum-bailiff' and a 'land-grabber'. The letter was supported by a couple of members of the committee, evidently also members of the United Irish League.[82]

The new order in Irish asylum management was signified equally by the innovations in the Cork district after 1900. A dominating figure on the Cork asylum committee was Bishop Kelly of Ross. It was he who drafted a plan for the conversion of the disused industrial school at Youghal into an auxiliary asylum for the Cork district. From 1900 to 1905 a battle raged between the articulate and determined Bishop Kelly, backed by his committee, and the inspectors of lunatics, with some support from the medical profession. The inspectors' attitude to the plan, suspicious in the first place, was hostile in the extreme when the committee decided to appoint a lay manager and give the running of the institution to a community of nuns. The inspectors saw the committee going

> back on the legislation and practice of the last half century which ... placed over the certified insane in all Institutions, medical men to be responsible for the patients' treatment, both as regards their bodily health and mental condition.[83]

Yet the inspectors' attachment to the wisdom of medical supervision proved less compelling than Bishop Kelly's arguments for a 'wider' view of the matter. The Youghal asylum, he told Sir Antony MacDonnell, the Under-Secretary, was only an 'incident' in his policy:

> I wanted to relieve the congestion in the main asylums by transferring the harmless patients to Auxiliary Asylums—to lighten the burden on the Local Taxation [Account] and thus keep it solvent ... and at the same time to lighten the burden on the local rates.

If the government did not concede to the Cork committee the right to establish a non-medical asylum on the grounds of economy, he

believed there would be much resentment of Dublin Castle in Cork.
This, a persuasive point for the Under-Secretary, would be a bad thing
for the government as 'the evil reputation of the Castle was beginning
to subside'. The question, Kelly was arguing, was not one which
related only to the care of lunatics and idiots.

> The inspectors in Lunacy have no idea of, or concern with,
> anything but the responsibility towards the idiots; and indeed the
> Inspectors never struck me as having statesmanlike breadth of
> view. But His Excellency, Mr Wyndham and yourself *must* take a
> higher and wider, and a more far reaching view of the matter.[84]

In the end 'higher' considerations won out against the vehement
opposition of the inspectors; the Youghal asylum was established with
a non-medical manager, but under the control of the Cork superintendent
'in the last instance'.

This episode is highly instructive. In a new political context the
balance of power in the asylum system *could* be shifted away from
medical control. But the failure of other asylum committees to adopt
this solution to the problem of overcrowding (a statutory solution
under section 76 of the Local Government Act) shows us that this
course was not an easy one. It was Kelly's energy and commitment to
what was, in fact, a social policy for Ireland which provided the drive
in the Cork situation. As he told MacDonnell, the 'greater part of my
life has been spent in the care and management of Institutions—
colleges, schools, infirmaries, hospitals and Asylums—as chaplain,
teacher, manager, governor and chairman of Boards'.[85] While there
were plenty like him eager to steer Irish education in a certain
direction and others keen to see land reforms, there were few
individuals on asylum committees before or after 1898 prepared to
commit much time to a consideration of how Ireland could best
provide for its insane. As his letter implied, however, even this
consideration was in the context of the wider sphere of politics and
self-determination. The important point was respect from Dublin
Castle for local authorities' ability to solve their own problems.
Elsewhere, for instance, Bishop Kelly argued *against* an increase in
the Treasury grant on account of lunatics; the money required should
be raised out of Irish resources, by increasing the local taxation.[86]

For the most part the promotion of alternative policies was foreign
to the reformed asylum committees. Passive resistance and symbolic
gestures to demonstrate that something was being done to lessen the

rates were more characteristic. After 1900 nothing less than half a million pounds was being spent annually on asylum maintenance and repayments. What committees could not do in the way of reducing the cost of provisions, they might attempt by refusing to build extensions or cutting doctors' salaries. The latter became a common enough action in the early years of the century. Just as dispensary doctors increasingly had to be satisfied with a lunacy (committal) fee of one pound instead of two, so asylum superintendents saw their salaries dwindle and the government ineffective in resisting this. Applications by superintendents at Cork, Letterkenny and Enniscorthy for increased salaries in view of their increased administrative duties under the Local Government Act were refused; the Mullingar committee opposed the appointment of a second assistant medical officer on the grounds of expense.[87] When superintendents died or retired the committees took the opportunity to reduce the salaries for new appointees—at Maryborough from £450 to £300, though restored to £350 after a protest from the Castle; at Cork, Monaghan and Carlow the committees followed the Maryborough example when new appointments came up.[88] The Monaghan governors consented to raise the salary after intervention from the inspectors who cited the opinion of the 'Lords Justices' that the amount they had fixed was inadquate.[89] Of course, such measures had little effect on asylum budgets and some committees (or the county councils behind them) grew resistant to embarking on any new capital works. The Sligo asylum in particular was chronically overcrowded yet neither Sligo nor Leitrim council would vote money for its improvement; no doubt part of the reason was that the district was already paying the highest rates in Ireland for the support of lunatics (9·3d in the pound, as against the national average of 5·6d in 1903-4). Although the committee had wanted to spend £45,000 on new buildings in 1900, the request was rebuffed by both councils.[90] By the time the Monaghan committee agreed to carry out additions in 1904 the sleeping rooms had almost double their quota of beds and nearly all had patients sleeping on the floors.[91] Yet the inspectors had trouble convincing not only asylum committees, the taxpayers' representatives, but even commissioners of inquiry about the urgency of the situation. The viceregal commission on poor law reform even remarked on the superiority of asylums to workhouse hospitals; the commissioners implied that the important thing was to raise the standards of care of the sane sick to those of the insane.[92] In this atmosphere the resistance of asylum authorities to increased expenditure must have won

considerable public support.

Apart from the resistance we have just described, the characteristic response to increasing problems with asylums was a revival of the call for a state take-over. In 1902 the councils of County Cavan, Belfast Borough and County Dublin all urged the government to bear the total cost of lunatics. In 1903 and again in 1906 the Ballinasloe asylum committee urged the same and in the latter year were supported by the Letterkenny, Mullingar and Castlebar committees.[93] There was, of course, a degree of ritual involved in the passing of these resolutions; but there was also a lot of support for the idea and not just from taxpayers. The inspectors of lunatics themselves had favoured the transfer to state administration. They cited the precedent of some of the United States and the British colonies. Their opinion, given to the royal commission on local taxation in 1899, differed substantially from that of the English and Scottish commissioners in lunacy who considered that public opinion was against centralisation.[94] This interesting divergence between Irish and British opinion on the question of nationalisation was repeated in 1907 when the Irish branch of the Medico-Psychological Association forwarded a number of resolutions to the government advocating a more effective lunacy department and various amendments to the lunacy law and administration. The memorial concluded that a strong case could be made out for converting the asylum service, like the poor law medical system, into a national service. The central body of the association, meeting in London a month later, approved of the resolution with 'the slight exception of the last paragraph', that is the one dealing with the nationalisation of the asylum service.[95] But, if there was any pressure building up from the joint forces of asylum committees and superintendents, it abated quickly enough. There was no indication that the government was going to increase the Treasury grant or deal with Irish asylums especially. On one side, the future of Irish government was in the balance with the Liberals promising home rule. On the other, the royal commissions on the poor law and on the feeble-minded (neither of which dealt in depth with the Irish situation) necessarily meant the delay of any comprehensive rearrangement of the asylum question in any part of the United Kingdom. So the nationalisation of the asylum service was left to another day.

The failure of these relatively *ad hoc* alternative policies— auxiliary asylums, increased government finance, nationalisation— left in the end only passive resistance. The increase in admission and residence rates led, by 1911, to the exhaustion of the local taxation

account—from then the local rates had to take a greater share of the burden.[96] This provided an even stronger motivation for resisting central direction. It was not surprising that the Irish insubordination to the 'jurisdiction of the lawfully constituted authorities', noted by Inspector Courtenay in 1901, was widespread among asylum committees by 1911. Hence, when the government attempted to legislate for the control of asylum-staff working conditions in 1911 the inspector of lunatics (T.I. Considine) questioned whether there was sufficient authority in Ireland to compel the committees to observe the regulations.

Experience has shown that there is under the present condition of affairs, the greatest difficulty in compelling the local authorities to carry out their existing duties as regards making provision for the insane, and in point of fact, if they take up a determined attitude, they can practically set the law at defiance.[97]

A number of asylum committees opposed the Bill and put pressure on local members to oppose it, on the grounds of the increased expense involved in reducing working hours.

The stalemate which had developed in the years after local government reform was characterised finally by the failure of the mental deficiency legislation for Ireland. As we have implied throughout this chapter, the question of a policy and practice for the care of lunatics and idiots was in Ireland subordinate to the broader concerns of Irish self-determination and the problems of local taxation. So when the royal commission on feeble-mindedness was appointed in 1904 it was not to be expected that its concerns would be equally shared in Ireland as in England or Scotland. The 'feeble-mindedness' question owed its prominence to the broader context of eugenics, national efficiency and social reform. But eugenics was not an important or contentious issue in Ireland; its ideology and its sometimes drastic solutions to the social evils it identified were irrelevant to the problems of Ireland. Doubtless the religious culture of the Catholic majority in the country was also a stumbling-block to the consideration of the eugenic programme to control the fertility of certain classes by abortion and sterilisation. Clearly it is of some significance that the only branch of the Eugenics Education Society in Ireland was located in Belfast.[98]

Thus the royal commission was only minimally concerned with Ireland. Its witnesses there, all of whom stressed the urgency of

special insitutions and education for idiot children, were professional men — the inspectors of lunatics, asylum medical officers and some prisons administrators. There was little doubt in the minds of the commissioners that the care of idiots, or mental defectives as the new terminology had it, was more desperately required in Ireland than in Britain. But there was no evident public demand for it; there was little concern with the implications, as the eugenists painted them, of a failure to deal with the problems of feeble-mindedness; and there was the problem of the asylum committees and the county councils which were opposed to any further expenditure. Consequently, when the Liberal government brought in a Mental Deficiency Bill in 1912, some four years after the commissioners' report, Ireland was not included in its provisions.[99]

The matter was not left there. Naturally enough there was support from some quarters in Ireland for this Bill which would encourage the establishment of special institutions for defectives. The Irish division of the Medico-Psychological Association protested at Ireland's exclusion; several MPs (three Unionist, two Nationalist) in the Commons in June and July supported Ireland's inclusion.[100] Birrell, the Chief Secretary, told the House on 15 July that the Bill would apply to Ireland. But there were troubles within the Irish party and opposition within Ireland to it. Birrell wrote to John Redmond on 30 July stressing the urgency of getting agreement from the Irish representatives so that Ireland could be included in the financial provisions of the Bill.[101] But agreement was not forthcoming in 1912, nor in 1913 when the Bill was enacted. The explanation of this failure is virtually a summary of what had happened to the asylum system in Ireland after 1898.

Undoubtedly the most important reason for opposition was financial. By enjoining local authorities to provide appropriate accommodation for certified pauper defectives, even with the aid of a government grant, the Bill was hardly appealing to local authorities which had suffered an abatement in the grant from the exhausted local taxation account in the previous two years. The inspectors of lunatics, though very much in favour of the Bill, were from the start sceptical of its potential in Ireland where, they noted, 'great difficulty is experienced in inducing local authorities to fulfil their existing obligations'.[102] Some local bodies did support the Bill—the asylum committees at Down, Cork and Waterford for instance. And there was predictable support from Irish branches of the National Society for the Prevention of Cruelty to Children and the Belfast branch of the Eugenics

Education Society. But probably more typical of public opinion was the Dublin corporation's support for the extension of the measure to Ireland 'provided that the cost of administering it be borne by the treasury'.[103] The Treasury would be contributing to the costs but certainly not paying all. A meeting of the Monaghan and Cavan asylum committee in July 1913 decided to seek the opinion of the local MPs. One favoured the Bill; the other two said the financial arrangements were inadequate and that it would impose a serious burden on the rates. The committee endorsed the latter opinion.[104] With lack of agreement from the Irish members, Birrell decided not to introduce the Irish clauses.

Finally, there was another consideration which was at play in determining whether this was a suitable measure for Ireland. The introduction of the Mental Deficiency Bill was preceded in England by widespread public lobbying. In fact, two private Bills were already before the House when the government brought its own measure in— one had been sponsored by the National Association for the Care of the Feeble-minded and the Eugenics Education Society; the other by the Charity Organisation Society. This expression of interested opinion, we have already suggested, was absent from Ireland. In fact, there was some feeling within the bureaucracy that the ascertainment and certification of defectives by magistrates would not be warmly received. The inspectors warned of this in their observations on the Bill and a memorandum by the registrar in lunacy for Ireland (J. Colles) agreed with them.

> It must be remembered that although in England eugenics have for years been the subject of discussion and legislation, such topics have been little ventilated in Ireland; and while specialists are agreed as to the gravity of the situation, the present proposals are not unlikely to startle and alarm unprepared public opinion in Ireland, if the administration of the Act is not handled with the utmost prudence and sympathy. To attempt administration on the lines of police regulation is to court failure.

If the Bill was to be extended to Ireland, both the inspectors and the registrar wanted to see justices specially appointed for the purpose of the Act, not the resident magistrates against whom there was 'prejudice in some districts'.[105]

By 1912 then, it was evident that the context of Irish public opinion had to be carefully assessed in the formation of social policies for

Ireland. The asylums which nearly a century before had been established as part of an administrative plan for the amelioration of Ireland were no longer seen as an enviable legacy of the Union. The existence of the insane, when noted, was resented as a heavy burden on limited local and national resources. The balance of power had tipped from Dublin Castle to popularly-elected local government authorities. With this change the emphasis of asylum politics shifted, from the mid-century obsession of the inspectorate with confining *all* the insane, to the provincial preoccupation of the early twentieth century with reducing numbers of inmates and certainly costs. The interests of the confined themselves were largely ignored in the course of this shift of power. Yet confinement of all who could be identified as insane was in itself a problematical policy. The fate of the lunatic will be our concern in the following chapters.

Notes

1. *JMS*, vol. 32 (1886), p. 22.
2. See Appendix, Table B.
3. *Hansard*, 4th ser., vol. 152, 183 (19 February 1906).
4. *Journal of Psychological Medicine*, vol. 4 (1851), pp. 257-9; *Hansard*, 3rd ser., vol. 114, 733-5 (17 February 1851).
5. *JMS*, vol. 7 (1861), p. 324.
6. J.L. Hammond, *Gladstone and the Irish Nation* (Cass, London, 1964) (reprinted), p. 95.
7. D. Thornley, *Isaac Butt and Home Rule* (MacGibbon and Kee, London, 1964), pp. 63-4.
8. A copy of Lambert's memorandum, prepared at Gladstone's instruction, is in T.H. Burke Papers, Bundle No. 3, SPO, Dublin. On Lambert see R. Lambert, *Sir John Simon 1816-1904* (MacGibbon and Kee, London, 1963), pp. 524-6 and R.M. McLeod, *Treasury Control and Social Administration* (Bell, London, 1968), pp. 8, 11-14. In 1867 Lambert had reported (very favourably) on the Irish medical service, *Report on the System of Medical Relief to the Out-door poor in Ireland ... HC* (1867), lx. He was later involved in a major capacity in the preparation of the Irish land legislation of 1870, E.D. Steele, *Irish Land and British Politics* (Cambridge University Press, London, 1974), pp. 137-8. Some reform of the local taxation system was achieved through the 1870 Land Act which set the country cess for all *new* agricultural lettings on the same basis as the Irish poor rate, W. Neilson Hancock, 'Local Government and Taxation in Ireland' in J.W. Probyn (ed.), *Local Government and Taxation* (Cobden Club, 1875), p. 220.
9. Thornley, *Isaac Butt and Home Rule*, p. 176.
10. *Hansard*, 3rd ser., vol. 210, 1331-48 (16 April 1872). The motion had a majority of 100 against the government. On Lopes and the local taxation question see Paul Smith, *Disraelian Conservatism and Social Reform* (Routledge and Kegan Paul, London, 1967), pp. 132, 207-8.
11. *Hansard*, 3rd ser., vol. 218, 653-8 (16 April 1874). Smith, *Disraelian Conservatism and Social Reform*, pp. 257-9 questions whether the Conservative government's measures can be dignified with the name of a 'policy' and sees them

instead as piecemeal, empirical measures largely dictated by the times.

12. *26th Report*, p. 10, *HC* (1877), xli; see also *25th Report*, p. 9, *HC* (1876), xxxiii.

13. RP 1899/13720, 1890/12151.

14. RP 1874/10160, 1874/10506, 1874/11333.

15. See Appendix, Table D.

16. RP 1899/13720, 1890/7756.

17. Cf. R.D. Crotty, *Irish Agricultural Production: Its Volume and Structure* (Cork University Press, 1966), Appendix, Table V, p. 356.

18. See Appendix, Table C.

19. *Freeman's Journal*, 31 January 1873.

20. *Report of the Select Committee ... on Grand Jury Presentments*, p. 59, *HC* (1867-8), x.

21. *MPC* Irish Supplement, 8 July 1874. Cf. *MPC*, 24 June 1874 and 20 August 1874 for Waterford demands for ratepayers' representation.

22. A select committee sat through three sessions (1876-8) and a viceregal commission of inquiry was also conducted in 1877 in an attempt to find the basis for reform, or at least compromise. James Lowther's Bill, introduced in February 1878, would have empowered reconstituted county boards (half-elected by cesspayers) to nominate two-thirds of the governors of asylums. *Hansard*, 3rd ser., vol. 238, 507-14 (28 February 1878).

23. *Hansard*, 3rd ser., vol. 262, 1483 (28 June 1881).

24. RP 1887/10943.

25. *Freeman's Journal*, 17 November 1887.

26. RP 1889/20780 includes an analysis of the city's grievances.

27. RP 1890/16262.

28. Cf. J. Morley, *Recollections*, vol. 1 (Macmillan, London, 1917), pp. 338-40.

29. *Hansard,* 4th ser., vol. 8, 311 (2 February 1893) (J.A. Rentoul, Down East); for a similar view of the 'Morley magistrates', see C.P. Crane, *Memories of a Resident Magistrate 1880-1920* (T.A. Constable, Edinburgh, 1938), p. 191.

30. *Hansard*, 4th ser., vol. 8, 337-8 (2 February 1893); for Unionist opposition to the new boards see ibid., 230 (2 February 1893), 301 (2 February 1893), 401 (3 February 1893), 523 (6 February 1893), 876 (9 February 1893).

31. Cf. Catherine B. Shannon, 'The Ulster liberal unionists and local government reform 1885-98', *Irish Historical Studies*, vol. 18 (1972-3), pp. 407-23; L.P. Curtis, *Coercion and Conciliation in Ireland* (Princeton University Press, Princeton, 1963), pp. 381-7; F.S.L. Lyons, *The Irish Parliamentary Party, 1890-1910* (Faber, London, 1951), pp. 67-8.

32. 61 & 62 Vic., c. 37, s. 4; ss. 9, 58 dealt with lunatic asylums.

33. Curtis, *Coercion and Conciliation in Ireland*, p. 386.

34. RP 1898/11428, 1898/8005, 1898/7180.

35. *Hansard*, 4th ser., vol. 57, 101 (2 May 1898), 116 (2 May 1898); vol. 58, 51 (18 May 1898). See also ibid., vol. 64, 123 (4 August 1898) for similar comments during the supply debate in 1898.

36. See correspondence in the Larcom Papers, NLI, Naas to Larcom, 16 February 1859 and Larcom's reply, 8 March 1859, MS. 7775/93-4.

37. Nugent to Fortescue, 19 January 1869, 20 January 1869, 7 April 1869, 6 May 1869 in T.H. Burke Papers, Bundle No. 3, SPO.

38. RP 1889/8232. This was, of course, true of the responsibilities of inspectors in many areas of the Victorian administrative structure in Britain and Ireland. The essential difference in role was between those who were significant innovators (in the case of this study, Francis White) and those whose activities were restricted to an essentially routine administration of their departments (Nugent and Hatchell). On the nineteenth-century inspector in Britain see D. Roberts, *Victorian Origins of the British Welfare State* (Yale University Press, New Haven, 1960) and Oliver MacDonagh, *A*

Pattern of Government Growth, 1800-1860 (MacGibbon and Kee, London, 1961), pp. 332-4.

39. RP 1861/9629.

40. Joseph Hatchell was at Maryborough, George Hatchell at Letterkenny.

41. Cf. *24th Report*, p. 217, *HC* (1875), xxxiii.

42. RP 1873/12945; the *Medical Press and Circular*, November 1872 to April 1874, carries extensive coverage of the Danford case.

43. The Attorney-General regretted that Fitzgerald could not be brought to trial; see letter from C.P. (Pallas, the Attorney-General) 6 December 1872, T.H. Burke Papers, Bundle No. 3, SPO.

44. *MPC*, 27 May 1874.

45. RP 1906/990, 1877/1083.

46. RP 1906/990, 1873/5231.

47. RP 1889/8232.

48. RP 1879/19809.

49. RP 1878/10404; cf RP 1860/12232, for a similar case.

50. RP 1889/8232.

51. RP 1882/47295. The dispute centred on Nugent's interference with Lalor's responsibilities. Extraordinarily, Lalor had been excluded from the board meetings since 1871 but Nugent attended the board until 1882. For the details and the inquiry, RP 1883/3273, 6130, 10243, 30859 and 1906/990.

52. RP 1883/17018.

53. RP 1887/13281.

54. RP 1906/990, 1887/13281, 1885/2004, 1885/12294.

55. RP 1889/8232 details the background to the inquiry.

56. Ibid.

57. *First and second reports of the Committee appointed by the Lord Lieutenant of Ireland on Lunacy Administration (Ireland), HC* (1890-1), xxxvi (hereafter *Mitchell Committee*).

58. Biographical details from the Kirkpatrick biographical files, RCPI Library, Dublin and *JMS*, vol. 36 (1890), pp. 309-10; O'Farrell had been the doctor required to report on the condition of John Dillon in Kilmainham gaol, 1888, F.S.L. Lyons, *John Dillon: a biography* (Routledge, London, 1968), pp. 98-9.

59. *JMS*, vol. 36 (1890), pp. 309-10.

60. RP 1890/10738.

61. RP 1906/2070, enclosing a report by the inspectors for the Chief Secretary on the defects in lunacy administration in Ireland, 31 October 1893.

62. *MPC*, 9 July 1890.

63. *40th Report*, p. 14, *HC* (1890-1), xxxvi.

64. Ibid., pp. 22-4.

65. Ibid., p. 202.

66. *Hansard*, 3rd ser., vol. 345, 715 (12 June 1890) and vols. 346, 1610 (12 June 1890).

67. *41st Report*, pp. 6-8, *HC* (1892), xl.

68. RP 1906/2070. Capital costs of asylums had originally been financed by interest-free Treasury loans, repayable over a period of 14 years; from 1877 (under the Public Works Loans (Ireland) Act, 40 & 41 Vic., c. 27) interest was charged on these loans.

69. *43rd Report*, pp. 13-14, *HC* (1894), xliii; Public Works Loans (3) Act of 1893, 56 & 57 Vic., c. 65, s. 1.

70. RP 1896/11927; *Hansard*, 4th ser., vol. 42, 1108 (9 July 1896).

71. *44th Report*, pp. 11-14, *HC* (1895), liv.

72. 38 & 39 Vic., c. 67, s. 9; *44th Report*, p. 18, *HC* (1895), liv; RP 1887/13281 for Richmond asylum's practice of discharging inmates to the South Dublin workhouse, under s. 11, freeing the asylum of financial liability.

73. RP 1891/17162.

74. RP 1912/4077, inspectors' minute, 22 March 1901. Ironically the Richmond asylum's boarding-out proposal arose from the difficulty of finding a suitable building for conversion to an auxiliary asylum, the establishment of which had been urged by the inspectors to solve overcrowding in the North Dublin workhouse lunatic wards.

75. R.B. McDowell, *The Irish Administration* (Routledge, London, 1964), p. 159.

76. *MPC* 8 September 1880.

77. RP 1896/19217, 1897/18677, 1898/8992.

78. *Hansard*, 4th ser., vol. 152, 183 (19 February 1906). There is a wide-ranging literature on the domestic concerns and reforms of Edwardian Britain. See in particular Bernard Semmel, *Imperialism and social reform* (Harvard University Press, Cambridge, 1960); G.R. Searle, *The Quest for National Efficiency* (Blackwell, Oxford, 1971); J.R. Hay, *The origins of the Liberal welfare reforms 1906-1914* (Macmillan, London, 1975); Anna Davin, 'Imperialism and Motherhood', *History Workshop*, vol. 5 (1978), pp. 9-66. For the Irish scene compare Lyons, *Irish Parliamentary Party* or David W. Miller, *Church, State and Nation in Ireland 1898-1921* (Gill and Macmillan, Dublin, 1973). Irish unionism, as opposed to nationalism, was primarily defensive in nature and its first interest was of course political. The ultimate failure of 'constructive unionism' is symptomatic of the difficulties faced by those who sought social and economic reforms in an attempt to solve the country's political problems. See F.S.L. Lyons, *Ireland since the Famine* (Fontana, London, 1973), pp. 202-3.

79. F.S.L. Lyons, *Irish Parliamentary Party*, pp. 253-4.

80. RP 1899/10300 (cutting from *Irish News*, 6 June 1899).

81. RP 1904/8809.

82. *MPC* Irish Supplement, 6 March 1907 (Ballinasloe); RP 1901/6531 (Sligo).

83. RP 1909/22928, encl. 1901/4302.

84. RP 1909/22928 (Kelly to MacDonnell, 11 October 1903).

85. Ibid.

86. See his evidence before the *Vice-Regal Commission on Poor Law Reform in Ireland*, ev. 28537 ff, *HC* (1906), lii; also *Conference of Irish Asylum Committees* (1904), pp. 102-7. In 1911 Kelly was to take a similar stand on old age pensions, arguing that Ireland, under home rule, would be unable to afford a pension system on the English model; the net would have to be drawn 'more tightly'. David W. Miller, *Church, State and Nation in Ireland*, pp. 278-81.

87. *MPC* Irish Supplement, 4 December 1901, 8 and 21 January 1902, 1 November 1905.

88. Ibid., 19 July 1905, 26 September 1906, 6 February 1907, 29 May 1907.

89. Ibid., 6 February 1907.

90. *53rd Report*, p. xxxii, *HC* (1905), xxxv; RP 1903/24426.

91. *53rd Report*, p. 137, *HC* (1905), xxxv.

92. *Vice-Regal Commission*, para. 159-62, *HC* (1906), li.

93. RP 1906/8307.

94. RP 1907/12449; *Royal Commission on Local Taxation*, Appendix, pp. 185-7, 193-7, 204-5, *HC* (1900), xxxvi.

95. RP 1907/12449. Irish medicine was historically more amenable to concepts of 'public' or 'state' medicine and thus, as in this case, less alarmed by the spectre of 'nationalisation'. For one thing the majority of the profession was engaged in public service through the dispensary system. Potentially the state could be seen as liberating doctors from the control of poor law guardians or, in the case of asylum 'doctors', from committees of management. On the tradition of 'State Medicine' in Ireland see R.M. MacLeod, 'The Anatomy of State Medicine: Concept and Application' in F.N.L. Poynter (ed.), *Medicine and Science in the 1860s* (Wellcome Institute of the History of Medicine, London, 1968), pp. 210-11. There is a useful summary of the 'public' status of the Irish medical profession in the preface by A.H. Jacob to R.J. Kinkead, *The Guide for Irish Medical Practitioners* (Dublin, 1889). Jacob pointed out that 1,051 of

the 1,800 practising doctors in Ireland were employed in the poor law medical service. A further 68 were in the public lunatic asylums: the latter, he believed, were 'entrusted with the control of the asylums to an extent not normal in other Civil Service Departments'. Ibid., pp. x-xi.

96. See RP 1911/442. As a result of increasing payments out of the Local Taxation (Ireland) Account, principally for lunatic asylums, the Irish government had to reduce the capitation grant to each asylum by 32 per cent in 1910. As John Dillon had warned in 1898 the relatively static amount of revenue from licence duties was thus shown to be quite inadequate to meet local needs.

97. RP 1911/18919.

98. See *The Eugenics Review*, vol. 3 (1911-12), p. 373 for the formation of the Belfast branch. For the opposition of Catholic teaching to compulsory sterilisation (for example in the papal encyclical *Casti Conubii*, 1930) see John T. Noonan, *Contraception. A History of its Treatment by the Catholic Theologians and Canonists* (Belknap Press of Harvard University Press, Cambridge Mass., 1965), pp. 430-1. Noonan refers to a later period than we are dealing with but it seems likely that Catholic social policy before the First World War would emphasise care of the feeble-minded rather than control of their propagation by means of surgical intervention. G.R. Searle, in *Eugenics and Politics in Britain 1900-1914* (Noordhoff, Leyden, 1976), pp. 13, 113, notes the consistent opposition of Catholics to eugenics from the very start of the movement. Certainly it is well known that in Ireland in the 1940s and 1950s the Catholic hierarchy was strongly opposed to a proposed national health scheme which the bishops regarded as impinging on areas of 'sex relations, chastity and marriage' in which the state had no right to interfere. See J.H. Whyte, *Church and State in Modern Ireland 1923-1970* (Gill and Macmillan, Dublin, 1971). For the Catholic Church's role in encouraging a very ascetic attitude towards sexuality in Ireland, see the argument of K.H. Connell, 'Catholicism and Marriage in the Century after the Famine' in his *Irish Peasant Society* (Clarendon Press, Oxford, 1968).

99. See *Royal Commission on the Care and Control of the Feeble-minded*, ev. 22080-23271, for Irish evidence, *HC* (1908), xxxvii. See also the reports of this commission's special medical inquiries on the incidence of, and status of care for, the feeble-minded in Ireland (Dublin, Cork, Galway, Belfast), *HC* (1908), xxxviii.

100. RP 1919/25489; *Hansard*, 5th ser., vol. 39, 1314; vol. 40, 52, 1157 (17 June 1912).

101. RP 1919/25489.

102. Ibid. (Considine to Dowdall, 17 June 1912).

103. Ibid.

104. *MPC*, Irish Supplement, 16 July 1913.

105. RP 1919/25489. For the background to the act see K. Jones, *A History of the Mental Health Services* (Routledge, London, 1972), pp. 191-8; and Harvey G. Simmons, 'Explaining Social Policy: The English Mental Deficiency Act of 1913', *Journal of Social History*, vol. 11, no. 3 (1978), pp. 387-403. Nikolas Rose has analysed the development of psychology in relation to its place in the social administration of the feeble-minded in 'The psychological complex; mental measurement and social administration', *Ideology and Consciousness*, vol. 5 (1979), pp. 5-68.

3 THE LAW AND THE INSANE

Developments in the law were as profound in their implications for the insane in the nineteenth century as the foundation of the asylum itself. Legal observers spent much time discussing the problem of lunacy and its relation to crime.[1] Yet of far more significance socially and economically was the process whereby thousands of people were confined in public asylums in Ireland, Great Britain and elsewhere.

In this process the law (its statutes and its instrumentalities) had a crucial role to play in Ireland. Yet it was one which was relatively unnoticed when compared to the lengthy debates over the 'criminal lunatic' and his actions in the pages of the medical, legal and social inquiry journals. Occasionally (in England and Scotland more often than in Ireland), the adequacy of the law would be called into question in relation to committals to *private* asylums, but hardly ever in relation to *public* asylums. The poor had few enough defenders, and the lunatic poor even fewer. A Charles Reade might discover an abuse in a private asylum, encourage legal action by the victim, then appropriate the case for a popular novel; but he was tapping deep-seated fears about the convenient committal to a private asylum for reasons of pecuniary gain. It was an appeal to the middle class in defence of the middle class.[2] But what was said about the practice of certification of 'private' lunatics might just as well have been applied to the much greater number of 'public' lunatics. In England there was, after 1853, one good legal reason why the committals of the poor attracted little attention: most committals after that date were outside the judicial system, were in fact part of the poor law administration. The same can be said of Scotland. In both cases, the role of the law was therefore obscured. But in Ireland certification at petty sessions was the most important mode of admission to district asylums. In Ireland, therefore, the law was not only central to the provision of asylums (in the sense that they were statutory institutions); it was also the primary determinant of the population of asylums. The instruments of the law, the magistrates, the police and in this case the doctors, defined what madness was and appeal against their decision was rare.

In the following account we will consider three aspects of the law in its relation to insanity and the insane: first, the history of the law of judicial committal in Ireland in the nineteenth century, as well as the

companion modes of admission to public and private asylums; secondly, the administration and practice of the law, its use in the hands of magistrates, police and doctors; finally, the constraints the lunacy laws placed on individual liberty and what protection, if any, the law gave to the rights of those who had been certified.

'Dangerous Lunatics'

Some aspects of the English background are pertinent in considering the history of judicial committal in Ireland. Outside the special case of chancery, which dated back to Edward II, lunacy was ignored by the law prior to the eighteenth century. It is well known that lunatics were restrained, if at all, along with petty criminals, vagrants, the destitute poor, in poorhouses and houses of correction. Indeed it was under the vagrancy laws that the statutes first attempted to control the lunatic. The Vagrancy Acts of 1714 and 1744 distinguised a class of 'furiously mad' or 'dangerous' persons who might be committed by two or more justices of the peace to a 'secure place'.[3] Section 20 of the 17 Geo. II of 1744 demonstrated the uncertainty with which this new class was defined, and that the innovation was a matter of public order; thus the justices were empowered to order the apprehension of

> Persons who by Lunacy or otherwise are furiously mad or are so far disturbed in their Senses that they may be dangerous.

Interestingly, and perhaps surprisingly for such an early statute, the clause also implied that the lunatic should be maintained and treated, though what was meant, beyond restraint, is unclear.[4] The 1744 Act empowered local authorities to board out the detained lunatics in private 'madhouses'. It is likely that it thus contributed substantially to the expansion of these houses in the later eighteenth century.[5]

While these Acts of the eighteenth century specified measures for the control of the insane, their context was the control of the vagrant poor. It was not really until 1800 that the statute law was directed to the control of lunacy itself, separately from the problem of the lunatic poor. The critical event of that year was, of course, the attempt of Hadfield on the life of George III. When his lawyer successfully argued Hadfield's defence on the grounds of insanity the government responded with legislation for the 'safe custody of insane persons charged with offences' and for the judicial arrangements in future

cases of insanity pleas. If, as Walker has suggested,[6] the courts had been faced with an increasing number of insanity pleas since the 1760s, and was treating them more sympathetically, then the Hadfield case was merely the catalyst for the legislative change. However that may be, the greater significance of the Act as far as the insane generally (not just those who had committed crimes) were concerned was its 'preventive' clauses. For 'the better Prevention of Crimes being committed by Persons insane', section 3 enacted that a justice might commit any person

> discovered and apprehended under Circumstances that denote a Derangement of Mind and a Purpose of committing some [indictable] Crime [as] a dangerous Person suspected to be insane.[7]

In such a case, bail could be set only by two justices or a higher judge. There was no mention in this Act of criteria of insanity, nor was there provision for medical evidence; indeed the only requirement was a suspicion of insanity. This was the basis of the later Irish Act and of similar statutes in the British colonies. In its failure to delineate procedural safeguards against subjective judgements and in its application to a person's *potential* actions the Act was initiating substantial constraints on individual liberty.

In the absence of public asylums for the insane, the persons committed under section 3 of the 1800 Act were sent to gaols. Considering the arbitrary powers given to magistrates under the Act, it is somewhat surprising that more extensive use was not made of it. In 1807 in the county of Middlesex there were only seven lunatics in gaols and twenty-seven in the houses of correction.[8] Even so, their alleged disruption of prison discipline provoked some discussion of their future confinement. Indeed the presence of lunatics in gaols offended the principles of separation and classification which were the backbone of the prison reform programme. And it was the Gloucestershire prison reformer, Sir George Onesiphorus Paul, who wrote a detailed and sophisticated submission advocating special provision for lunatics in public asylums for the 1807 select committee on criminal and pauper lunatics.[9] In spite of the hesitant start on the provision of public asylums in the following years, it was not until 1838 that Parliament made it possible to send 'dangerous lunatics' to asylums, indeed to prevent them being committed to gaols in England.[10] In the same session of Parliament, the first Act dealing with the confinement of 'dangerous' lunatics in Ireland was passed.

Strangely, although Ireland already had a system of public lunatic asylums, this Act instituted the now anachronistic English practice of sending the insane to gaols.

Prior to 1838 there had been, as we have already seen, a number of statutes dealing with the accommodation of lunatics in Ireland and with the detention of criminal lunatics. The former matter, involving as it did extensive state intervention for the construction of asylums, has been examined in Chapter 1. But we should note that the important Act of 1821, which established the public system, provided that criminal lunatics—those acquitted on grounds of insanity at the time of the crime, or found insane at the time of indictment—would be detained in the lunatic asylums at the pleasure of the Lord-Lieutenant.[11] This was the opposite of the English practice before 1838, which confined them in gaols. As for the mode of admission of non-criminal lunatics, the Act of 1821 made no provision, leaving it to regulations at a later date. The early practice was admission by order of the board of governors on application to them by a relative or friend of the alleged lunatic (or another 'interested person').

The Dangerous Lunatics Act, passed in the first year of Victoria's reign, was retained in its essentials well into this century. The details of the passage of the Act are obscure, since no debate was reported on it. However, the circumstances were in large part similar to those of the 1800 English Act. It was introduced following the murder of a 'most respectable gentleman' (the words of the inspector of lunatics) in Dublin by a man who had been refused admission into the Richmond asylum a short time before.[12] Like its English predecessor of 1800 (and indeed its companion of 1838) the Irish Act made 'Provision for the better prevention of Crime being committed by Persons insane'. By 1838, however, the assistance of medical evidence was considered important. Any two justices of the peace were empowered 'to call to their Assistance any legally qualified Physician, Surgeon or Apothecary' in the case of any person 'apprehended under Circumstances denoting a Derangement of Mind, and a Purpose of committing some [indictable] Crime'; if, on examination of the person 'or from other proof', they were satisfied that he or she was a dangerous lunatic or idiot, the justices could commit the person to gaol. There the person would remain until discharged by an order of two justices (including one who had signed the committal warrant) or until removed to a proper lunatic asylum by order of the Lord-Lieutenant.[13] Two features of the Act are worth comment. One is that while medical evidence could be called for, the

justices were free not to do so and to make the commital on their own judgement or even 'from other proof', that is the statement, not even sworn, of some person who sought the committal. As yet medical opinion was dispensable. Secondly, there is the curious fact of the committal being made to gaol in the first instance, with perhaps a transfer to an asylum at a later stage. Why a practice which Parliament had legislated against for England was instituted for Ireland in the same session is not at all clear. Two factors may have been considered in the drafting of the Bill. Although there was a national system of public asylums, there were at this stage only ten asylum districts. Many of these covered very large areas—the Ballinasloe asylum served the whole of Connaught, the Limerick asylum all of Counties Clare, Kerry and Limerick. Thus it may have been considered that a preliminary and readily available detention in a local prison was preferable to a journey of some days to the district asylums. Secondly, by requiring the Lord-Lieutenant's warrant, the Act instituted some central control over asylum admissions, a control which might be needed in case of overcrowding or too many committals under the new Act. The former was probably the dominant consideration.

Besides this form of judicial committal, which became the most important mode of admission in Ireland, there were other ways of being confined as a lunatic. For public asylums, the most important of these was an application to the manager by a relative or friend of the person involved. This had to be endorsed by a magistrate or clergyman to the effect that the person was poor enough to be entitled to public care, together with a medical certificate testifying to the person's insanity. This application would be considered by the manager and the physician of the asylum before being put to the asylum board for acceptance. As well the rules for the 'Government' of public asylums, approved by the Privy Council in 1843, provided for admission by the physician in cases of emergency. This provision was only one of a number of innovations which in 1843 had given medical men a pre-eminent role in Irish asylums.[14] It was also to prove a loop-hole in the system of control of admissions by the asylum board—by the 1870s the asylum superintendent, rather than the board, was authorising the great majority of the 'ordinary' admissions.

For private asylums, relatively insignificant in Ireland, an Act of 1842 provided that all admissions should be at the instance of an order made out by a relative or friend. In this case, however, the admission required certificates from *two* doctors who had separately examined

the 'Patient'.[15] This requirement had its origins in the English agitation over private madhouses. The distinction in the practice of certification between private and pauper lunatics (that is two doctors versus one) reflected the fundamentally different histories of the two classes. Public asylums ('district' in Ireland, 'county' in England) were founded with the paternal object of care of the insane poor; thus only one certificate was required, it being assumed that no advantage, other than a social one, would accrue to the partners in the committal of a poor person. Private asylums, on the other hand, had an infamous reputation as places where profit was made out of madness and where wealthy people might be shut up to the pecuniary advantage of their relatives: two medical certificates were thus deemed to be necessary protection against abuse. However, as far as the law was concerned, both public ('ordinary') and private admissions were of similar status—they were admission orders only and were not, in fact, legal for detention of the person confined as some doctors later found out to their loss.

During its thirty years' existence the Dangerous Lunatics Act created a series of crises for both the asylum system and the prisons to which the 'dangerous lunatics' were committed in the first place. From the beginning it appeared that committal under the Act could be obtained quite easily. Indeed, as we have seen, the law left it open for a person to be committed on an information which was not taken on oath or recorded. There were neither safeguards for the liberty of the individual nor against the law's own misuse. It was the strength of criticism on these grounds by an 1843 House of Lords committee and by asylum boards in response to the report of that committee which led to an amendment in the law in 1845.[16] Section 10 of the 8 & 9 Vic., c. 107 (the statute which created a separate lunacy inspectorate) required that a person not be committed as a 'dangerous lunatic' without an information on oath of one or more credible witnesses given before the committing justices. Under the amendment this information was to be forwarded to the clerk of the crown or clerk of the peace, a provision which was mandatory but not always carried out. In August 1847, two years after the passing of the Act, the inspectors of lunatics drew the attention of the Under-Secretary to irregularities in the committal procedure, including the failure to forward copies of the sworn depositions to the clerk. Consequently, large numbers of cases were committed to gaol for indefinite periods without an opportunity for reviewing their condition: the inspectors evidently considered that it was at least their business, if nobody

else's, to undertake such a review. It was not even clear from their inquiries how many people had been committed to gaols under the 1 Vic., c. 27, but of the 368 they could locate, 40 per cent had been in prison longer than one year. Failure to call for a medical opinion during the judicial examination (this was not mandatory) was also widespread—173 of the 368 committals did not have a medical certificate. Following the inspectors' report, the Under-Secretary circularised magistrates urging their caution in the use of the Act. A year later the government, at the inspectors' prompting, issued a standardised warrant of committal, hoping that this would engender a greater compliance with the legal forms. From another angle, the inspectors sought to ensure that all committals of lunatics to prison came under their notice by proposing the establishment of a 'Central Registry of Criminal and Dangerous Lunatics'. This innovation was also adopted—from November 1847 gaol governors were asked to forward the details of all committals to the lunatic asylums' office.[17] Thus, through these bureaucratic devices, the inspectors managed to bring the fairly indiscriminate detention of lunatics in prisons under some control. Ten years later, when a royal commission obtained a return of the dangerous lunatics in gaol, less than 20 per cent had been there longer than twelve months, a considerable change from 1847.[18]

However, these attempts to exert control over magisterial behaviour and to refine government knowledge of the committals were not, in the long term, adequate to resolve the problems caused by the Act. For relatives or friends, there were considerable advantages in the use of judicial procedure rather than the ordinary mode of admission. For example, the usual form of admission to an asylum required an engagement on the part of a responsible person to take back the lunatic when called on to do so by the asylum board. Use of the Dangerous Lunatics Act avoided the need for this commitment. By making the person in essence a 'criminal' lunatic the judicial procedure entailed a public responsibility for his maintenance. This opened the door, so some believed, to the not-so-poor, and even to the well-off, to commit lunatic relatives to the gaol, from where they would be transferred to the district asylum.[19] Formally the asylum was open only to the poor, that is, according to the Cork admission form, those unable to afford a private lunatic house. The Kilkenny asylum board complained in 1861 that by such a practice an injustice was done to the poor for whom the institution was intended.[20] Doubtless, they also thought an injustice was being perpetrated on the ratepayers. Yet the weight of this objection was probably exaggerated. The inspector of lunatics,

George Hatchell, agreed with the Kilkenny board and claimed that there were at least 66 patients in Irish district asylums who were capable of paying maintenance but had been committed as dangerous lunatics. But these 66 were only a fraction of the 5,000 resident in asylums in 1861. This sort of objection sounded plausible enough but the figures hardly suggest a major abuse in this area.

A true picture of the use of the Act was, in fact, very hard to obtain. Besides claiming that some relatives used the law to avoid maintenance charges in private asylums, the inspectors blamed the families who allegedly instituted committals to 'get rid of the care and support of their insane relatives' or even of those merely troublesome 'from old age, bad temper, physical infirmities and the like'.[21] While such a charge had the support of asylum governors, we do have the contrary evidence of one who was rather closer to everyday practice. A Dublin magistrate who dealt with large numbers of these committals denied that relatives wanted to commit lunatics to avoid future financial liability for them or that they wanted to get rid of them in any way possible. In the first place, he pointed out, he could not 'recollect a lunatic being brought before [him] whose friends or relatives appeared to be in a state even of respectability'. Most committals were obviously of the very poor who would be quite incapable of contributing maintenance anyway. Yet he had often found that

> persons charge lunatics in the expectation that they would be sent to an asylum, and that when they found that our first committal was to a common gaol, they have over and over declared that out of their earnings they would try to pay something if the person could be sent to an asylum at once.

They did not wish them to be subjected to the degradation of a prison.[22] As we shall see in the following chapter, the relatives of lunatics were not always as benign in intention as this account suggests. But it does qualify the position taken by the inspectors that the families of the insane poor were ever ready to deposit their relatives elsewhere.

Besides these 'social' reasons cited as an explanation for over-use of the Act and therefore grounds for reforming it, there were criticisms of the legal system and its irregularities, and questions of the statute's institutional impact on prisons. The root of the problem, according to the inspectors, was the carelessness of magistrates in the practice of committal. The magistrates not only neglected to make proper

inquiries into the cases brought before them (which allegedly made it difficult for doctors to treat the insane) but would 'not infrequently sign committals without ever having seen the lunatic at all'. In nine cases out of ten, the inspectors claimed in 1864, one justice alone saw the lunatic, the second signing the committal as a matter of course. Elsewhere they estimated that one in every five or six committals was irregular. In some cases justices, who were also guardians, were said to be committing the troublesome inmates of workhouses to asylums, people who might have 'smashed a window' or 'torn a pillowcase'.[23]

The feeling against the Act among those other than the inspectors related more to the alleged harm done to lunatics in gaols, and the indiscipline occasioned by their presence, than to the faults of magistrates. In 1843 Lord Monteagle thought the ill-effects of imprisoning lunatics in gaols self-evident. There were other considerations besides those of humanity, he told the Lords—how could gaols be 'properly governed' when they had fourteen or fifteen lunatics in them?[24] Twenty years later an Irish MP urged the assimilation of Irish lunacy law to English, to allow magistrates to commit dangerous lunatics to county asylums:

> lunatics were not efficiently looked after in gaols, and the discipline of the gaols was much interfered with by having lunatics there, and the difficulty of management was increased.[25]

The confinement of lunatics in gaols had long been criticised and condemned. It was an easy point to bring against an anachronistic Act in the 1860s.

It is evident from all this that there was hardly a word to be said in favour of the first Dangerous Lunatics Act. Why, then, was it not amended earlier? Only five years after its enactment, the committal of lunatics to prisons was condemned by the Lords committee on the state of the lunatic poor in Ireland.[26] Similarly the royal commission in 1858 recommended a change in the law.[27] And with the constant criticisms by the inspectors in their annual reports an earlier amendment might have been expected. Two reasons for the failure to amend the Act until 1867 seem relevant. One was the question of the asylum system's capacity to take all the committals which could be made by magistrates. In the 1840s it was already clear that considerable numbers were being refused admission to the district asylums for want of room. During the 1850s and 1860s the government directed a very substantial expansion of the system, to

accommodate the potential lunatic population. While this expansion was going on Dublin Castle was reluctant to change the law and thereby put pressure on the existing asylums: Sir Robert Peel (the Chief Secretary in the early 1860s) defended the *status quo* by arguing that the government was doing all it could to expand the asylum system; when six new asylums were completed all the 'criminal lunatics' in gaols would be committed to them.[28] As well, while the inspectors were the strongest critics of magisterial practice they did not want to see justices (of whom there were some 3,600 in Ireland) given power to send lunatics direct to asylums. Since magistrates already sent so many to prison (the inspectors cited an extravagant estimate of 800 to 1,000 committals per annum, whereas the average was about 700) 'they could at once set about clearing the localities in which they reside of any person who could be at all considered as affected with mental disease'.[29] While the inspectors exaggerated the case it was at least true that committing to asylums rather than gaols would double the number of dangerous lunatics eventually sent to asylums. Already in the early 1860s over 25 per cent of all admissions to public asylums were by judicial committal and a change in the law could be expected to raise this to over 40 per cent.[30]

The second reason for the failure of an earlier amendment was a political one. In fact, Lord Naas had attempted in 1859 to enact some of the recommendations of the royal commission, including the assimilation of the English practice by which relieving officers of the unions were responsible for arranging lunacy committals. But this Bill failed hopelessly, not because of this innovation but because of the more contentious and absorbing issue of local control over asylums. The fact was that what political energies went into the Irish 'lunacy question' in the 1850s and 1860s were centred on the problems of taxation, local control and the placement and construction of new asylums—issues we have examined previously.

Nevertheless, it was Lord Naas himself who was finally responsible for the Bill amending the old Act, brought in on 9 July 1867. It stopped the 'barbarous practice', as he put it, of confining lunatics in gaols, empowering justices to send them to district asylums instead. The previous system had not proved 'beneficial or desirable' and 'the presence of a number of these prisoners rendered it impossible to carry out the proper discipline of the prisoners'.[31] There was little debate reported on the Bill, and none at all on the adequacy or otherwise of the judicial committal procedure. Yet it was this, rather

than the English practice, which the new Act enshrined. For one reason or another the English procedure, using the poor law system, was not adopted, as it had been in the 1859 Bill. The most likely explanation is that the system of care of the lunatic poor in Ireland was quite distinct from and preceded the Irish poor law system. The two were much closer administratively in England and the prime consideration—the taxation base—was different in the two countries. To have the confinement of the lunatic poor (who were maintained on the county rates in Ireland) administered by the relieving officer was considered inconsistent. The use of dispensary medical officers as the certifying doctors in the committal procedure was not inconsistent since the intention of the dispensary system was relief of the *poor* who were sick, not just the destitute.

Hence the new Dangerous Lunatics Act treated the lunatic in substantially the same way as the old. Two justices, as before, were empowered to commit 'Dangerous Lunatics' or 'Dangerous Idiots' to district asylums—but it was now incumbent on them to obtain a medical certificate from the medical officer of the dispensary district in which they were sitting.[32]

Dublin Castle was well aware at the end of 1867 that the new Act might place great strains on the asylum system. In an attempt to pre-empt a rush of committals to asylums, the Chief Secretary issued a circular to magistrates on 30 December. They were advised of the changes in the law and urged to observe the importance of obtaining evidence of a purpose of committing an indictable offence. The experience of the previous thirty years suggested the need for a more insistent caution. Magistrates were advised that they should only exercise their powers under the Act against persons likely to commit acts of violence and crime. This warning was not enough to allay the fears of the inspectors of lunatics who advised asylum superintendents the following day to arrange for the transfer of 'quiet and harmless lunatics' to workhouses. In this way, they hoped, there might be room in overcrowded asylums for the new committals.[33] Yet, as one would expect, this particular gambit was not welcomed by the poor law guardians; the poor law commissioner, Alfred Power, attacked Nugent's attempts to influence the management of workhouses in this area; and the government legal officers thought it was probably illegal to solve the asylums' problems in this way.[34]

Before long it was clear that the inspectors' worst fears about increasing committals would be confirmed. One of them reported to the Under-Secretary on 3 February that there had been seven

committals to Armagh asylum in January 1868—there had been only one in the same month the year before.[35] A week later the board of governors at the same asylum complained about the overcrowding caused by the reception of dangerous lunatics since the beginning of January. Moreover, these committals were made with such vague and unsatisfactory information about the lunatic that the board requested a new warrant—the government prepared and issued this later in February. Early in March it took further action to secure, in the words of T.H. Burke, the Under-Secretary, 'a proper administration of the Law'. Asylum superintendents were asked to inform the inspectors of committals made under the old form (the 1838 Act), or failure to give all the information required; the poor law commissioners were asked to draw the attention of dispensary doctors, who were responsible for medical certification, to the necessity of special personal inquiry in each case; and the inspectors of lunatics were to report improper committals to the Lord-Lieutenant.[36]

No doubt the official attempts to control, or at least to regularise, the judicial process on the magisterial bench met with varied response. In 1869, two justices at Listowel considered the evidence insufficient to commit a workhouse inmate to the asylum. They

> would willingly have sent the case to the Asylum but that they have been sent Circulars directing them to be more cautious in sending to the Asylum only such cases as they shall be satisfied are dangerous lunatics.[37]

But such caution was not exercised in the same degree elsewhere. At least, so it was felt by some asylum administrators. The Omagh governors wrote of the great inconvenience of patients being sent to the asylum under the new Act. They wanted the government to send a circular to magistrates and police officers in Fermanagh and Tyrone directing them not to send lunatics without prior communication with the superintendent of the asylum. This was rather more than the government felt it could do. The Omagh board was told that they should provide extra accommodation; their suggestion, a government official commented, was 'contrary to law and common sense'.[38] At another stage in the first year of the Act the Armagh governors attempted to control the crisis of overcrowding by directing the resident physician to write to magistrates asking them to inform him before committing lunatics. Again the government took a dim view of local interference with the legal process. The governors were informed

that warrants under the Act were mandatory and immediate.[39]

In spite of the attempts by central and local authorities to minimise the impact of the Act, it was quite evident by the end of 1868 that it had been widely, and probably loosely,used. The experience of the first year led the inspectors to believe that magistrates 'appear to consider every lunatic brought before them as "dangerously insane", and to issue a warrant accordingly'. Unfortunately we do not have judicial statistics available to tell us how weighty this charge was. There may well have been many more alleged lunatics brought up at sessions and *not* committed—the committal rate of the magistrates may have been just a reflection of a much greater use of the procedure by the public at large. However that may be, while 634 persons had been committed as dangerous lunatics under the old Act in 1867, 979 had been committed to asylums in 1868.[40] When committing to asylums, the magistrates were not exercising that caution in discovering the details of the case which they had supposedly applied in the past.[41] The result was 'indiscriminate committals of reputed "dangerous lunatics" '. Many exhibited no symptoms whatever to justify their committal—some were described as blind, crippled, helplessly paralysed, 'deaf and blind with great debility' and could hardly be considered dangerous.[42]

In the following years the inspectors continued to watch over the use of the Act and criticise its widespread application. Cases were frequently referred to them from the asylums; from the lunatic asylums' office some went to the government's legal officers for an opinion as to their legality. For some years one common failing was the use of the old warrant for committals to gaol. In spite of instructions to the contrary in 1869 and 1874, these warrants were still being used in parts of Wexford and Galway in 1883.[43] While, on one level, this was only a lapse in a matter of form, on another, it reflected the extent to which even elementary legal procedure could be ignored in a lunacy committal. Even after the Act had expressly prohibited committal to gaols the justices could disregard it. In the second year of the Act 149 lunatics were placed in bridewells from one petty sessions to another (perhaps eight to ten days, claimed the inspectors) while the justices made a decision about their sanity.[44] Even in Dublin where the frequency of cases should have made justices aware of the legal formalities, a warrant for committal to gaol was made out as late as 1899.[45] Irregularities in the form of committal were so frequent that an amendment (in the 1875 Lunacy Act) provided for the correction of a defective form within 14 days of

admission.[46] The defects in the warrants ranged from the examples
above to failure to state the required details of jurisdiction and the
occasional case where medical certificates were given separately
from the magistrates' hearing.[47] From the 1870s to the 1890s the
government frequently circularised magistrates and petty sessions'
clerks in order to regularise magisterial practice.[48] However, by 1897
Dublin Castle intervention was less acceptable. An inspector of
lunatics agreed to a request by the local government board in that year
for magistrates to be informed that committal of dangerous lunatics to
workhouses (they referred to a case in Castlerea union) was illegal.
But he was overruled by the Assistant Under-Secretary who told the
board that it was not the practice to advise magistrates as to the
discharge of their duties—specific cases would be dealt with as they
came up.[49]

Whatever the inspectors were able to achieve with individual
magistrates the administration of the whole of Ireland was obviously
beyond them and the statistics demonstrate the increasing use of
judicial committal over time. Table 1 demonstrates that there was a
greater use of the procedure from the first available figures (which are,
of course, gaol committals) to the turn of the century. During the
1850s and 1860s dangerous lunatics constituted less than half of
'public' lunatic admissions. By 1890 the authority of the Dangerous
Lunatics Act was behind three out of four male admissions and nearly
seven out of ten female admissions. Thus it had become the routine
mode of entering the asylum.

Table 1: Committals of Dangerous Lunatics as Percentage of Admissions to District Lunatic Asylums

	Male	Female
1854-6	41·8	31·8
1860-2	49·8	34·7
1870-2	56·9	43·3
1880-2	62·5	48·0
1890-2	75·7	67·3
1900-2	72·3	60·2
1910-2	76·2	58·8

Note: The 1854-6 and 1860-2 figures are for comparison only and have
been calculated as though all committals to gaol under 1 Vic., c. 27 were
instead sent to asylums.
Source: Annual reports of the inspectors of lunatics.

In general, as the figures in Table 1 make clear, it was applied more often to men than to women. Perhaps this phenomenon reflects a greater difficulty in controlling intractable males outside the asylum and, conversely, a tendency for any female violence to be neutralised within the family. Equally it might arise from the susceptibility of males to prosecution for drunkenness, a more commonly cited 'cause' of insanity among male inmates than females.[50]

The Act was not enforced to the same extent in all asylum districts. As Table E (Appendix) shows, in some areas the Act was much less commonly used than the national figures would suggest. Local variation was most obvious in the first year of the Act, 1868, when one asylum (Sligo) recorded no admissions under judicial warrant while another (Armagh) received nearly 90 per cent of its inmates that way. The Sligo case was unique and probably the result of an arrangement between the asylum superintendent and local magistrates, or merely of a very flexible admission policy. All but two of the seventy admissions to Sligo asylum in 1868 were 'cases admitted by the Resident Medical Superintendent as "urgent" '. During the previous year the practice was similar—only one lunatic had been committed to Sligo gaol in 1867, certainly the lowest incidence of such committals in the country. Within a couple of years, however, Sligo had become typical of the rest of the country in using judicial committals. The relative importance of the Act as it applied to men and women also showed important regional variations. In some areas, Monaghan and Letterkenny, for example, there was little distinction made in applying the Act to men or women; in Belfast and Down, however, it was used mainly against males. Without detailed study of a number of particular areas it would be impossible to determine the weight of factors responsible for these local variations within the national trend. Obviously admission policy at the asylum was probably important—as asylums became overcrowded superintendents probably resisted 'ordinary' admissions. Monaghan, for instance, was extremely overcrowded from the 1880s and the Dangerous Lunatics Act provided almost the exclusive mode of admission in that area. Beyond this institutional factor, however, the use of the Act is buried in the unquantifiable depths of magisterial, police and medical attitudes and practices and not least in the complex area of the social context and behaviour of lunatics.

Thus an Act which was intended primarily for the prevention of criminal offences became the major mode of committing the insane. In spite of constant allegations of its misuse the Dangerous Lunatics Act

survived beyond the end of the Union in 1921. This was certainly not through a desire on the part of policy-makers and bureaucratic guardians of the insane to perpetuate it. Hardly a year went by without the inspectors complaining publicly (in their annual reports) of the anomalies of the Act and the great burdens it imposed on the district asylums; and their opinion, of course, was not the only source of opposition to the Act. Asylum doctors, though not unified in their attitude, were frequently critical. Dr Oscar Woods of the Killarney asylum regarded the Act as inflicting an injury on the lunatic by branding him as criminal, an injury which also affected his friends. On the public, he said, it also had the undesirable effect of 'breaking down those strong barriers which ought always to separate visitations of Providence from vicious acts'.[51] Similar in sympathy though concerned with quite another issue, was the attack on the mode of admission of the poor insane by Dr Garner of Clonmel asylum in 1878. He regarded both the dangerous lunatic's warrant and the 'ordinary' form of admission as defective since the certificate of only one physician was required in each case. For private (that is paying) patients, whether admitted to public or private asylums, two certificates were required. He considered it just as important to guard against improper detention of a pauper as of an individual 'in a higher social grade'.[52] The Mitchell committee felt the same way in 1890. Recommending a system of reception orders for all patients, it criticised the Irish system: 'Class lunacy legislation should so far as possible be avoided.'[53] However, not all asylum managers were convinced of its disadvantages. Questioned by the Trench commission in 1878 Dr Robertson of the Monaghan asylum considered it had not been frequently abused and that it encouraged the admission of patients in a 'more recent stage of insanity' (when, the orthodoxy held, it was more curable). Similarly, Dr Lalor of the Richmond asylum in Dublin denied that there was much abuse of the Act and thought it was well administered by the Dublin magistrates. But he did think that it was sometimes used in 'spite or spleen'. As well, because it was left to private initiative (a relative or friend in most instances), it was occasionally not used when it ought to be.[54]

Dr Lalor's last objection pointed to the most commonly proposed alternative to the Irish law. This was that the insane should be subject, as in English law (under the 16 & 17 Vic., c. 97 of 1853), to local inspection and committal through the poor law machinery. The amendment of the Act on these lines was recommended by the commissions of inquiry in 1858 and 1878 and formed part of Lord

Naas' unsuccessful Lunacy Law Amendment Bill in 1859. In the 1870s assimilationists such as William Neilson Hancock urged the introduction of an English-styled lunacy law before meetings of the Statistical and Social Inquiry Society of Ireland.[55] Yet, in spite of the efforts of this society's 'Charity Organisation Committee', parliamentary moves to amend the Irish law were singularly unsuccessful. Lord O'Hagan, one-time Irish Attorney-General and a member of this committee, introduced amending legislation several times with no result. To him in 1881, there appeared to be a 'scandalous indifference' on the part of the legislature and the country to the provision of institutional care for harmless imbeciles and idiots.[56] As O'Hagan's charge made clear, attempts to change the law drew their justification from the need to spread the legal net in order to institutionalise the harmless as well as the 'dangerous' insane. Such an alteration in the law would have had the effect of reducing the incidence of judicial committal. At the same time it would almost certainly have raised asylum admissions overall. And in involving the poor law machinery, the amended law would have increased the poor rates. This consequence was not lost on local authorities. When the government itself attempted an amendment in 1883 local opposition quickly forced the withdrawal of the Bill.[57]

The failure of both private and government attempts to amend the law in this period perhaps made later governments reluctant to undertake a major reform of the lunacy laws. This was unlike England (where a major overhaul of the law had taken place in 1890) and in spite of the weight of expert opinion against the existing law. As we have seen in Chapter 2, the administration of asylums drifted into stagnation after the 1860s and the Dangerous Lunatics Act survived for much the same reasons. If the procedure made 'criminals' out of lunatics there was little evidence that most people were disinclined to use it on that ground. And in spite of the frequent cases of irregular committals being referred to Dublin Castle, the attitude of the bueaucracy could be resigned. The solution advocated by a government law officer in 1876 was to call the attention of individual magistrates to particularly bad cases and 'to discharge a few for the sake of example'. He doubted whether any system not liable to abuse could be devised.[58] This was not the opinion of the inspectors of the medical profession nor of the Mitchell committee members, all of whom continued to advocate the amendment of the law.[59] But what we have already said about the failure of the mental deficiency legislation for Ireland in 1912-13 applies equally to the failure to amend the

Dangerous Lunatics Act. The dominance of the taxation question ensured Irish opposition to any attempt to increase the burdens on the poor rates by encouraging the comprehensive committal of lunatics on the English model. And the fragility of social 'reform' in Ireland as compared with the national question meant that there was very limited support for an appeal against the Act in the name of humanitarianism or rationality. As a consequence the majority of asylum inmates in Ireland continued to be detained under the provisions of what was a very illiberal law. The judicial committal was, as the Mitchell committee's report pointed out in 1890, an order of indefinite detention. There was no mandatory review of the condition and status of a person detained under the Dangerous Lunatics Act. This, even more than the alleged 'stigma' of having appeared in a magistrate's court, was the most alarming feature of the law.

In the most substantial nineteenth-century account of Irish lunacy law, G.W. Abraham, a former registrar in lunacy, claimed that most of the patients in district asylums were 'largely, even principally' from the 'class of dangerous lunatics'.[60] But the 'dangerous lunatics' in Irish asylums were usually not dangerous to themselves or society. It was the peculiar survival of a law which had its origins in an attempted assassination of George III which constituted them dangerous.[61] In the following section we will consider in more detail the practice of the law's instruments, with a view to understanding the phenomenon of its increasing use in Ireland.

Police, Doctors, Magistrates

The lunacy laws required instruments of enforcement and in Ireland these consisted of the justices, the police and the doctors. We have already seen that magisterial practice was commonly criticised; that their administration of the law was frequently less than satisfactory and sometimes bordered on the illegal. That was the view from Dublin Castle. But their position was an ambiguous one—while finally responsible for a lunacy committal the actual role of the magistrates was probably subsidiary to that of the police, who had the job of arresting, conveying and restraining the person, and the doctors, whose certificates, based variously on careful or cursory examination, were the formal declaration of insanity.

It is, of course, impossible to imagine such a large-scale use of the

Dangerous Lunatics Act in Ireland without the creation, just prior to the 1838 Act, of the Irish constabulary. The establishment of this force, and of its predecessors going back to the late eighteenth century, took place in the context of widespread rural agitation, disorder and sectional conflict.[62] But once established, the force took on a wide range of responsibilities which extended its influence into many areas of Irish life. Thus, by 1859 a 'Constabulary Officer' could complain of the manifold duties imposed on the police. Among these he enumerated

> Revenue Police Duties; Enforcement of Fishery Laws; Suppression of Smuggling; Comparing Standard Weights and Measures; Billeting of Troops on March; Revision of Bridewell Books; Supervision of Petty Session Clerks' Accounts; Surveillance of Ticket-of-leave Convicts; Distribution and Collection of Poor Law Voting Papers ... Agricultural Statistics ... with many other minor duties, too numerous to mention.[63]

The multifarious duties of the Irish police constable included a certain responsibility for the care and control of lunatics. He had the obvious peace-keeping role entailed by the Dangerous Lunatics Act of 1838. While one might see this as a passive role—merely acting on the information of civilians—there were at least two ways in which their attention was directed towards active investigation of the lunatic population and its condition in society at large.

Occasionally police were directed by Dublin Castle to carry out benign investigations which might today be undertaken by a social worker. This might involve an inquiry as to whether a family would receive or maintain a lunatic or agree to a transfer to some other institution; or an investigation of allegations of neglect or ill-treatment of an insane person in family care.[64] Secondly, one of the other duties 'too numerous to mention' was the Irish census of lunatics at large, the administrative function of which we examined in Chapter 1. From 1845 to 1877 the constabulary was requested from time to time to take such a census of 'lunatics, idiots, imbeciles and epileptics' not in institutions. The returns were prepared in each sub-district and from 1856 specified the name, religion, residence and class of life ('Lower, Middle and Upper') of each insane person known in the area.[65] While the accuracy and utility of the survey was questionable by the mid-1870s, of greater importance was the fact that over a period of thirty years more than 6,000 potential inmates of asylums were known by

name and residence to the police. This knowledge signified the dramatic changes which had taken place since the turn of the century in the place of lunatics in the community. The state had intervened to establish institutions for the confinement and care of the insane poor. From relatively small beginnings with modest aims, the asylum system had expanded abundantly. In the course of this process the instruments of the law, the police in particular, had their attention directed not just to the 'prevention of offences by insane persons' (the object of the 1838 Act) but to the comprehensive knowledge of all insane persons in the community. When the metropolitan police superintendent could report in 1854 that the writer of an illegible letter sent to the Lord-Lieutenant was a 'lunatic named Philip Geoghegan who resides at Kingstown [and] is well known to the men of the G & F Divisions as such' he was demonstrating the arrival of the centralised and relatively efficient surveillance which the foundation of the Irish police had made possible.[66] The constable was instructed in his police manual to 'know if possible every person in [his] sub-district'.[67] It was the constable as much as the doctor and certainly rather than the magistrate who would know the insane at large in his area.

In relation more particularly to the *confinement* of lunatics the constabulary was indispensable. The constable could himself be the agent in the committal, in the course of maintaining public order. It was hardly an enviable task at the best of times; the police were no better equipped to understand or control a violent or agitated lunatic or drunk than the rest of the community and their intervention could itself be provocative. Thus, when Dr Norman of the Richmond asylum reported that a recent male admission had a fractured nose, allegedly after being beaten by a policeman, the constable concerned claimed he had been defending himself. He was not to know that Francis Dunne had just been prevented from cutting his throat by his brother. When he stopped him running down the North Circular Road at 1.00 a.m. with only shirt and trousers on, carrying his shoes tied together and his coat on his shoulder, he claimed that Dunne hit him in the face; in any case, a struggle ensued during which Dunne, according to the constable, fell on the footway. He took him to the police court next morning; after hearing the evidence, the magistrate called in a doctor who certified the man.[68] In the same way that they were responsible for controlling vagrants and drunks, police undertook the control of lunatics on the street.[69] An infraction of public order or a minor offence might be the cause of arrest but, in subsequent investigations, the police might call in the doctor, and then arrange a lunacy committal.[70]

There were other ways in which police could be actively involved in the control of the insane as defenders of the public safety. Thus numerous constables were directed to follow and watch 27 people discharged from Dublin gaols in 1845 after they were found to be illegally detained (on medical advice) as dangerous lunatics. Within a few days all had been retaken and newly committed.[71] Naturally enough, the surveillance of released lunatics was more commonly called for in the case of those who had committed criminal offences.[72] Akin to this duty was the role of the police in pursuing and retaking escaped inmates of asylums. The Lunatic Asylums (Ireland) Act of 1875 empowered asylum managers to retake an escaped lunatic without new certificates within fourteen days.[73] Sometimes asylum attendants were sent in pursuit of the fugitive but police were called in to follow any suspected dangerous person. Following an escapee's flight to America from Ballinasloe asylum in 1875 the inspectors undertook to prepare a standardised form for the description of escaped lunatics which superintendents would circulate to local police stations. They also suggested the insertion of notices in the *Hue and Cry* but the Under-Secretary queried this since the publication was 'intended for the arrest of *criminals*'. Evidently sceptical of the enthusiasm of his men for the pursuit of escaped lunatics, the inspector-general of constabulary suggested that a reward of one pound be paid to police for the arrest of each lunatic 'to encourage the Constabulary to read such notices and make these arrests'. But the Under-Secretary also overruled this, doubting whether such payments from asylum funds would be regarded by the auditors as having been made for the 'care and maintenance of patients'.[74] In any case a reward was probably unnecessary. Most escapees went back to their homes and were easily located by police or attendants. Of 32 escapees from Irish asylums in the three years to December 1888 only one had not been recaptured.[75]

Finally, quite apart from their own initiative, police were an indispensable part of the practical business of confining lunatics. It was usually they, though sometimes the doctors, whom the relatives contacted to arrange the committal; and once the person was taken to the police barracks, it was the constable's job to get the justices and a doctor to attend and commit. When the committal had been made it was the policeman, perhaps even two, who conveyed the lunatic to the asylum. This could be a trying journey over long distances, perhaps taking 24 hours or more,[76] and in many cases involved restraint and violence against the lunatic. Police were not very well equipped in temperament or training for these tasks and there were common

allegations of ill-treatment, even with fatal consequences, involving police handling of lunatics. *The Irish Constable's Guide* of 1880 spent some time instructing its readers in the proper mode of conveying lunatics to asylums, the expenses of which were supposed to be charged to grand juries.[77] But the responsibility for ill-treatment lay not only with the police. Indeed the wording of the instructions referred to above derived from a circular to magistrates of 1875—this (from the Under-Secretary) asked the magistrates to afford the police 'suitable facilities ... to take the most humane care of the afflicted under their charge' and suggested consultation with the certifying physician as to 'the care and custody of difficult patients'.[78] What 'suitable facilities' were provided after 1875 is not clear but there appear to be fewer complaints after this date. Still, only a few months later the Castlebar asylum superintendent complained to Dublin Castle about two constables escorting a lunatic to the asylum with a three-feet ash sapling 'to threaten' him.[79] And asylum doctors continued to be unhappy about the condition of some of their admissions—Christopher K., who was received in 'a very battered condition had been tied with a rope which left contusions in arm & back', complained 'with justice of treatment he received at the hands of police', a Richmond doctor noted.[80] It was the policeman's role in the committal of lunatics which was one part of the asylum doctors' opposition to the 'dangerous lunatic' procedure. But the constable's attitude and treatment was certainly no different from that of the layman and compared with some relatives may have been more restrained. Without chemical restraint the control of the violent insane involved a substantial degree of physical force, tying with ropes, sitting on them and so on—all measures which no doubt provoked more violence.[81]

Before 1868 it was not incumbent on magistrates, though it was generally the practice, to obtain a medical certificate for committal of a dangerous lunatic. From that date, however, the doctor's certificate was essential, whatever the evidence of informants, were they relatives, police or otherwise. Although the law stipulated otherwise, the customary course was for

the police to call on the dispensary medical officer to examine an alleged lunatic prior to bringing him or her before two justices, so that they may produce before the justices, when sitting, both the alleged lunatic and the medical officer's certificate, or to have the medical officer present to prove his certificate, and that he examined the alleged lunatic.[82]

It was the dispensary doctor alone who was empowered to certify a dangerous lunatic from 1868. Since the creation of the poor law medical system in 1853 it had been one of his duties as a salaried officer.[83] The reason for the exclusion of private practitioners by the 1867 Act is unclear but was probably intended to economise local expenditure. Previously medical men had sometimes been paid by a magisterial order out of grand jury funds.[84] At the same time such an exclusion of private practitioners could be seen as protecting the insane (or sane) from being certified for a fee: feeling ran deep in the nineteenth century against doctors making money out of madness. But whatever the reason for requiring dispensary doctors to certify 'without fee or reward' the policy was soon reversed under pressure from the profession. Section 14 of the Lunatic Asylums (Ireland) Act empowered justices to make an order on the guardians for expenses associated with the examination, including the medical evidence, up to a maximum of two pounds.[85] The Irish Medical Association, which later claimed credit for the amendment, encouraged doctors to press justices for the fee by gratuitously providing forms to be filled in by the magistrates.[86]

Two things are worthy of note in considering the dispensary doctor's role in judicial committals. The first and most important is that most doctors were no better educated in the complex world of 'mental disease' than anybody else. There was little interaction between the *asylum* medical staff and the profession at large (including dispensary doctors) and no education in psychological medicine before the 1870s at the earliest. Even after this such courses were rarely compulsory. So when most doctors signed lunacy certificates they were not doing so on the basis of their possession of a specialised knowledge of insanity but rather on the basis of their rising professional status and the successful assumption by a fraction of the profession of the care of the insane.

Even so, signing lunacy certificates could be a troublesome and dangerous business, particularly in the late 1870s and early 1880s when doctors in England were losing court actions brought by certified patients. Indeed, in 1878 the *Medical Press and Circular* believed that 'the majority of medical men have a great objection to signing lunacy certificates'.[87] And more advanced parts of the profession suggested in the early 1880s that state-appointed 'examiners in lunacy' should alone be empowered to certify. Thus Dr Thomas More Madden, a prominent Irish gynaecologist, advocated such a reform in 1884, believing that

a question of such importance should not be left to the arbitrary and practically irresponsible judgement of any two gentlemen who happen to be on the Medical Register.[88]

These criticisms were concerned principally with the certification of private patients. But the reservations expressed about the competence of private practitioners could be applied twice over to the certification of the poor insane. The dangerous lunatic committal did not require that magistrates examine the medical evidence and, in consequence, the certification was little more than a matter of routine.

The medical certificate tended to rely on the evidence of the informant and others rather than on the adequate personal examination which the statute implied. Some doctors were clearly not sure about what they were supposed to be doing in a lunacy examination and acted against their better judgement. A Maryborough surgeon-apothecary who 'had the greatest difficulty in signing the certificate' said that the man committed had no delusions 'but a man might have them and I not discover them'. The chief reason for signing the certificate

arose from the fact that Mr Sullivan was once a lunatic, and from the circumstances of the certificate which I saw was signed by a Kilkenny Doctor, who must have known him personally—coupled with the history Mr Mulhallen gave, but which Mr S— contradicted.[89]

This was an ordinary committal not requiring evidence of the lunatic being dangerous. But when the latter was required it could be quite cursory. A seventeen-year-old labourer was a 'dangerous lunatic' because 'he can't be kept at home—but wanders about'.[90] The medical certificate of Patrick Britt, committed to Clonmel asylum on the information of a policeman, described the case as 'mania', the symptoms as 'maniacal' and was otherwise devoid of evidence—the Clonmel staff could find no symptoms of insanity while he was in the asylum.[91] The 'facts indicating that the Patient is a Dangerous Lunatic' in another Omagh committal were that she 'has been in Asylum for years'.[92] While the law had attempted to inject some expertise into the committal process, the personnel who were supposed to possess that specialised knowledge which could tell sane from insane commonly showed themselves to be incapable or merely indifferent to the task.

On the other hand, the one piece of quantitative evidence we possess on medical certification practice suggests a considerable discretion exercised on the part of the doctor. Unfortunately we cannot tell with certainty what criteria Dr R.S. Ireland (the medical attendant to the Dublin Metropolitan Police) was applying in concluding that over one-third of the 2,300 people brought before the Dublin police court on the charge of dangerous lunacy between 1845 and 1856 were not insane. His practice may have been determined by institutional pressure (for example, from the local gaols and asylums wishing to restrict as far as possible admissions of lunatics). But any doctor who saw as many alleged lunatics as this had probably also developed an intuitive, even idiosyncratic, understanding of the borderline between sanity and insanity. To Dr Ireland, insanity apparently implied dangerous behaviour. Asked whether a large proportion of those brought before him had no appearance of insanity he considered that they had not. Yet his evidence confused insanity and dangerous lunacy.

> When a husband, or a wife, or a child becomes imbecile or soft in intellect without being a dangerous lunatic the wife has attempted to get the husband committed, or the husband the wife. It was an attempt to get rid of the party affected, which I resisted as much as I could.[93]

We should recall that the Dublin magistrate examined after Dr Ireland disagreed that relatives were over-anxious to get rid of their lunatic charges. In any case the doctor's evidence suggests that when he said 'not insane' he meant merely 'not dangerous', a social as much as a medical judgement.

The second aspect of the doctor's role was the contribution of medical practice to greater use of the judicial committal rather than the ordinary admission procedure. In an article on 'The Insane and the General Practitioner' the superintendent of the Enniscorthy asylum, Dr Thomas Drapes, stressed the serious nature of a lunacy committal in view of the stigma which attached to admission to the asylum. He was particularly critical of the lack of detail in medical certificates. But he also drew attention to the popularity of the magistrate's warrant over the house form. It was popular

> with the public ... because it saves relatives all expense in getting the patient into the asylum; they simply 'press the button', the

police do the rest; with medical men, because a fee is allowed for certification in warrant cases, whereas none is given in the case of the House Form.[94]

In the year ended 31 March 1906 807 medical officers received £3,226 in lunacy fees.[95] This was not a great amount, but some doctors received considerably more than the £4 average implied by this figure. In fact dispensary doctors were quite disparately favoured with lunacy business. Many dispensary districts recorded no lunacy committals while others returned a dozen or more annually, on the part of one doctor.[96] Some doctors were apparently unlucky enough to have districts in which no magistrates sat, and therefore no lunacy business could be had.[97] This was mostly accounted for by the lack of identity of judicial, police district and poor law boundaries. But allegations were commonly made that magistrates directed lunacy business to particular doctors by choosing to sit in particular dispensary districts.[98] Again, the granting of lunacy fees demonstrated the routinisation of the lunacy law. Although the law stated clearly that the maximum fee of £2 was to cover all expenses (including transport, police costs etc.) it was common practice from 1875 for justices to sign an order for the whole amount to be paid to the doctor, and even in some cases two guineas.[99] Although such large amounts may have been justified in some cases where the doctor had to make two or three journeys to the home of the lunatic or the police barracks,[100] the frequency of the claims upset the guardians who had to pay. In several court actions they resisted payment, unsuccessfully, and later tried to influence the justices to reduce the fees.[101] But it was not until the 1900s that the courts agreed with the guardians.[102] Meanwhile many doctors found it preferable to arrange a lunacy committal for their poor patients and receive a sizeable fee for it than to sign a 'house form' for a patient they had visited on a red ticket (issued by a guardian to a person eligible for poor law medical relief) and receive nothing at all. The struggle for fees for committal of the insane poor completely overshadowed the more serious aspect of the doctor's role in the process—the fact that medical men continued to certify the insane without any special training or qualifications to do so. We find the evidence of what certification meant in the government and hospital archives, not in the *Medical Press and Circular*.

If first police then doctors played the crucial roles in the committal procedure as we have suggested, the magistracy, which received most of the blame for loose administration of the law, was merely presiding

over a pre-determined and routinised process. However, the justices were not uniformly passive, nor always regardless of the letter of the law as the inspectors and others frequently charged. In response to Castle circulars we have already seen that two justices in Listowel refused to commit a man who was evidently not dangerous.[103] At Naas petty sessions in 1875 the doctor declared a woman insane, but not violent—the magistrates declared they needed proof of an overt act before committing an insane person (in fact the statutory requirement was only a *purpose* of committing an indictable offence).[104] A police magistrate refused to commit an invalid pensioner because 'there was insufficient evidence of an intention on the part of the patient to commit any overt act of violence'.[105] But to adequately assess the extent to which a lunacy committal was anything more than a formality one would like to have figures showing the proportion of persons brought up as 'dangerous lunatics' at petty sessions and *not* certified. Unfortunately the judicial statistics do not provide this information. Instead we are left with the impressionistic evidence that magistrates understood the law imperfectly to the extent that during some thirty years following the 1867 Act they were repeatedly advised by Dublin Castle to observe the requirements of the law. Irish magistrates were more likely to be challenged by doctors over lunacy fees than by the people they confined over the legitimacy of their committal. In spite of the warnings from Dublin, the magistrates knew they were acting 'for the safety of the Prisoner and the Public'[106] and the Dangerous Lunatics Act was there to be used towards that end.

Lunacy and Liberty

We have seen how lunatics were defined and processed by the law for admission to asylums. How they were discharged from those asylums and what individual rights they retained under committal are the subjects of our concluding comments on the law and the insane. It must be noted at the outset that there were powerful forces at work constraining the rights of the insane in the paternalist defence of their welfare. Doctors were particularly inclined to wish away the legal obstacles in the path of treatment. Philanthropists and reformers in this area were also inclined to dismiss the queries which stood over certification and confinement. Lord Shaftesbury, anxious that his work for the insane should be safeguarded, hoped in 1880 that

nothing will be done which will throw unnecessary impediments in the way of early treatment by a mistaken delicacy in regard to the 'liberty of the subject'.[107]

The Director of the National Society for the Prevention of Cruelty to Children castigated the 'drivel' of one MP (probably Josiah Wedgwood) who had opposed the Mental Deficiency Bill in 1912 on the grounds of its invasion of freedom.[108] With supreme conviction that they knew what was right for the lunatic, reformers and doctors rarely conceded the necessity for questioning the process of committal and detention. In particular, when doctors were forced to consider the problem it was usually in the context of a spate of legal actions for false imprisonment: not surprisingly, their response was to look to legislative amendment to protect them in the future.

In examining this issue, there are two points to consider. One concerns the laws and regulations governing the discharge of asylum inmates, the other the status of lunacy certification at law, the prevention of false imprisonment and the actions open to individuals who considered they were wrongfully certified or detained. While it seems that it was only in England (if we are considering just the United Kingdom) that public opinion could be stirred to any great extent over these questions, the matter was not dormant in Ireland. A number of court actions highlighted the unique nature of lunacy committals and the peculiar extent of social control over the lunatic. There is little doubt about just how extraordinary lunacy certification was and is. A recent review of the law of habeas corpus notes the qualifications which have evolved to limit the right of habeas corpus of a certified person. This was a development in common law and statutes have not modified it. Thus one authority has written:

> The source of the power to refuse to discharge a person illegally committed simply because the court suspects he may be dangerous, is not at all clear. It seems to be assumed that there is an inherent sort of *parens patriae* jurisdiction which is exercisable to protect the interests of the public and of the patient. It is worth noting that, in balancing individual rights against the public interest, this kind of reasoning has never been openly applied in criminal cases where, very often, there is little doubt about the prisoner being dangerous.

As Sharpe goes on to note, there is the 'added consideration of the patient's interest which may not always be seen to allow for

release'.[109] What we will consider below has an important part to play in the delicate business of judging whose interests, the public's or the inmate's, the lunacy laws have served.

The manner of discharging a person from an asylum in Ireland initially depended on the mode of admission. The major distinction was between those committed as dangerous lunatics and those admitted otherwise. Under the 1838 Dangerous Lunatics Act those transferred from gaols to asylums by the Lord-Lieutenant's warrant (up to half of all asylum admissions before 1868) could be discharged only by order of the Lord-Lieutenant.[110] The criteria for discharge in the 1838 statute was that the person had become 'of sound Mind' and this was to be certified by two doctors. In 1845 an alternative criterion, that the person had ceased to be dangerous, was added.[111] In the following year the necessity of viceregal consent to the discharge of a 'dangerous lunatic' committed under the 1 Vic., c. 27 was removed.[112] Consequently, after 1846 the discharge of dangerous lunatics and 'other Lunatic Poor' was managed on the same basis. The formality was that the board of governors would discharge any inmate on the recommendation, by certificate, of the resident or visiting physician. This was the procedure ratified by the amended Act in 1867.[113]

Unquestionably such a system depended to a great extent on the initiative of the resident medical superintendent. Where the asylum was overcrowded there was some incentive in terms of management and health to keep reviewing the status of inmates. As well, a board conscious of the high costs of maintaining inmates in asylums, might well be anxious to discharge harmless patients to the workhouse. After 1867, however, discharge was not entirely dependent on the institution and its managers—section 10 of the 30 & 31 Vic., c. 118 empowered a relative or friend to take out an inmate, on entering into a bond 'for his or her peaceable Behaviour or safe Custody' before two justices. We should note here that there were no statutory provisions for reviewing judicially the status of an inmate, for giving him or her a right to investigation with a view to discharge. Beyond the medical officer, a relative, or a board member taking note of an inmate the only course open was a letter from the inmate to Dublin Castle. Responsibility for investigation would then rest with the inspectors of lunatics, both of whom were, of course, doctors. There was the possibility of legal action at the instance of the inmate or of an interested friend or relative. We will consider this course below. But first let us look at the question of a relative's application for an inmate's discharge.

Although the discharge 'on bail' provision of the Dangerous

Lunatics Act of 1867 appeared to be unqualified, asylum doctors
were already acquiring at the time substantial powers which would
eventually qualify that section. Thus in 1862 the Irish Attorney-
General advised Dr Lalor of the Richmond asylum that the board
could detain a patient admitted on the ordinary form, even after
friends or relatives had requested his release, if the medical officer
considered he was not fit to be discharged. The basis for this decision
was a Privy Council regulation of 1862 that no patient should be
discharged without a board order and the medical certificates of both
medical officers.[114] The opinion was substantiated in 1870 when the
law adviser noted that a man, who had, in fact, been released from
Castlebar asylum on the request of his father, might have been legally
detained if the superintendent did not consider him sufficiently
recovered. Following this case the inspectors of lunatics issued a
circular drawing the attention of asylum superintendents to their
power to detain a patient, admitted on an ordinary form, whose
release had been requested.[115]

In spite of this practice with regard to *ordinary* inmates (who
thereby seemed in a worse position than 'dangerous' admissions) no
attempt was made to test the right of release on bail of 'dangerous
lunatics' until 1894. Between 1868 and 1894 it was the practice to
hand them over to their friends upon the production of the recognisance
obtained before two justices. Thus, even though Dr Carre of Omagh
considered Eliza Stinson should not be released from the asylum in
1891, the inspectors and the law adviser warned him that section 10
was mandatory if adequate recognisance was produced; the justices,
the law adviser noted, were the judges of how adequate the bond
should be.[116] But in November 1894 the Court of Appeal in Dublin
held that the asylum superintendent had a discretion at common law
to decide whether a lunatic on whose behalf a recognisance had been
entered into should be discharged or not.[117] Thus it seemed that a
lunatic had only a limited right of habeas corpus, a point we will
examine later.

This was the position with regard to the release or discharge of
those not regarded as recovered or harmless. With respect to the latter
there was also a large amount of discretion in the hands of the asylum
board and superintendent. Regarding those who had recovered, the
law adviser in 1874 held that they could not lawfully be detained in an
asylum, even where they were not removed by their friends. Yet, in
fact, discharge was probably dependent very much on the prospects
for the recovered inmate outside the asylum, for instance, for those

who were useful workers in the asylum and without friends outside. As for those many inmates who were considered harmless, and for whom the asylum was chiefly a place of residence, the likelihood of their being discharged unless they had someone to take them was initially remote. Before 1874, indeed, the government law adviser could not see that the board had any power to discharge an incurable or harmless lunatic admitted on an 'ordinary' form. But an amendment to the Privy Council rules gave the governors the power to discharge a lunatic to his place of origin (this could be the home of those who had undertaken to remove him when recovered, or the workhouse) and recover the expenses of sending him there.[118] As these examples imply, the practice of discharge, quite as much as that of admission, was dependent on a complex of laws, regulations and local (both institutional and popular) opinion. The amendment we have just noted was in fact the product of a situation where asylum boards wanted to discharge inmates and could not because friends or the workhouse would not take them.

Finally, we should remember that although the board's consent to a discharge was in the main a formality, it did have the power to overrule the doctor's recommendation. In one sensational case the resident physician at Monaghan asylum certified an inmate, Father Mooney, as sane and ordered his discharge. But on the intervention of Bishop Donnelly the board of governors decided to defer the discharge 'on the understanding that the Bishop should have an interview with him'. The two asylum doctors were present at the interview and concluded that Mooney was still 'labouring under delusions' (which concerned the bishop himself) and was unfit for discharge. After some months, during which the government received various demands for an investigation into the case, the medical officers again found him 'much improved' and recommended his discharge to the care of his relatives.[119] In the absence of other evidence, one must conclude that such intervention by a governor of an asylum, against the recommendation of the doctor, must have been rare.

Such was the law and the practice of discharge of asylum inmates. What course was open to people detained in asylums, or their friends, to seek their discharge or discover the causes of their detention? We have seen already that there was no statutory judicial process of review or appeal against a detention. But the inspectors of lunatics did themselves have fairly extensive powers of investigation and the Lord Chancellor could direct them to investigate the case of any person

confined as a lunatic.[120] However, these investigations were dominated by medical criteria and the patient's liberties were usually qualified by these criteria. At one of the earliest of these inspectorial inquiries, Francis White used his powers under section 28 of the Private Lunatic Asylums (Ireland) Act to investigate the detention of William Cuthbert, a patient in a Cork private asylum. White considered some of Cuthbert's complaints, in particular his eight-year confinement in asylums, as justified and urged some measure of parole for him. Yet his fellow 'commissioners', three other doctors, disagreed with his lenient view and Cuthbert was not released.[121]

In attempting to use the inspectorial channels, inmates or ex-inmates or their friends could find themselves in a classic double-bind situation. It was, of course, the condition of admission to an asylum that somebody else signed the order or committal—an attempt to discover why this had been done, or who had done it, could render an inmate suspect of having delusions about continuing conspiracies. Thus, a request of Denis Linehan to see the documents relating to his previous committal in the Richmond asylum was opposed by the inspectors in 1878 in spite of the law adviser's sympathy with the request. Linehan, the inspectors explained,

> evidently feels him [sic] aggrieved for being placed in a Lunatic Asylum as if he were unjustly treated by the kindly intervention of his friends—This non-recognition of his past state of mind rather induces an apprehension with the Inspectors that he is not fully restored to reason.[122]

Once Dublin Castle, in the medium of the inspectors, had decided that a person's complaint was without foundation, it was considered better to ignore the letters: 'as the man is lunatic', concluded Thomas Larcom, the Under-Secretary, in 1853, 'it is better not to enter into correspondence with him'.[123] Some inmates at least were aware of the routine: in response to the persistent questions from one patient as to why he was sent in and why he could not be let out Dr Petit of the Sligo asylum

> advised him to write to the Inspector but he *smiled* at the idea, as he said, of writing a letter to the Inspectors which wd. be referred to me so that I might sit in judgement on my own action.[124]

The inspectors' attitude to the release of documents and the conduct

of inquiries depended not only on their judgement of the mental state of the complainant but also on the need to defend institutional and medical interests. Thus, after Nugent had uncovered a suspect certification in the confinement of a former mayor of Kilkenny, the inspectors seemed inclined to give details of their investigation to the man's solicitors but stopped at 'officially contributing information which may lead to litigation'.[125]

In the end, litigation was the only course if the inspectors refused to investigate or reported unfavourably on a case they had investigated. On occasion the government advised this course to dissatisfied inmates or their representatives, for example in the Cuthbert case, above, where the government told the man's solicitor to try habeas corpus. Under section 47 of the Private Lunatic Asylums (Ireland) Act, a writ of habeas corpus or other action against any person for confining an alleged lunatic obliged the former to justify the confinement according to common law. Of course legal action, whether habeas corpus or a suit against others for conspiracy, was expensive and was hardly open to most of the poor and even destitute inmates of asylums. Hence it was little used in Ireland and it was rare, relative to the enormous number of committals, in England. However, there were a number of cases of interest in establishing the limits of the alleged lunatic's liberty.

As we have previously remarked, the right of habeas corpus was considerably qualified in the case of lunacy committals. The Irish courts took much the same position as the English in the determination of this position. The following case, for instance, exemplifies the 'paternalist attitude' described by Sharpe[126] as determining the court's refusal to discharge a dangerous lunatic illegally committed. An action by the father of John Fetherstone, an inmate of the Clonmel district asylum, failed to obtain his release in 1860. The justices of the Queen's Bench in Dublin found that the magistrates who had committed Fetherstone as a dangerous lunatic had exercised their jurisdiction 'defectively and carelessly' to the extent that the committal was invalid. But with respect to the habeas corpus application the court decided to appoint medical examiners to determine whether Fetherstone was dangerous. Their report was that he was often violent and dangerous in the asylum; consequently the court discharged the conditional order for habeas corpus.[127] Perhaps it was this judgement which encouraged the practice, noted earlier, that even where a person had been admitted on an 'ordinary' form, the resident physician might refuse his discharge at a later date if he was then dangerous.

The condition on the right of habeas corpus was affirmed in 1894 when the Irish Court of Appeal ruled that there was no absolute right of a relative or friend to remove a lunatic from an asylum on recognisance. In their judgement the judges cited two English cases, one of 1846, the other of 1855, to establish that the court should consider whether the discharge of a person would be dangerous to the public or himself.[128] The courts considered that the detention of a person, while dangerous, was justified whatever the legal basis for the action. Hence, in 1868 the *Medical Press* reported a case where the jury decided that relatives, who had restrained a man who had committed acts of 'outrageous folly' and 'clear insanity' (evidently from the effects of drink), were justified in doing so; the judge had directed that a person should be restrained if dangerous to himself or others, but not if harmless.[129] Clearly this was the practice in the nineteenth century—the balance has tipped somewhat in favour of the alleged lunatic more recently and Sharpe cites a number of cases from the 1950s where the court discharged a person illegally committed *without* inquiry into his actual mental state.[130]

Nevertheless the law was ambiguous about lunacy detentions and the threat of legal action could hurry along a discharge. This was the reason behind Dr Courtenay's request to the inspectors to sanction the discharge of a nineteen-year-old girl in the Limerick asylum in 1879.

> The Father believes that his daughter was wrongly sent to the Asylum [she was committed from a convent]—cannot be made to understand that this is the proper place for her & is going about stating that his daughter is imprisoned against his wish.[131]

Where the person had not been committed as dangerous the certifying doctors and the person receiving the alleged lunatic (the superintendent or private asylum manager) could be vulnerable. A successful habeas corpus action at the Irish Queen's Bench in 1870 brought to notice that there was no defence for the superintendent of a private or public asylum against an action for unlawful imprisonment of a lunatic, unless certified as dangerous. Section 99 of the English Act, 8 & 9 Vic., c. 100, allowed superintendents to plead the ordinary lunacy certificates as justification for the confinement. Subsequent to the 1870 case, the man discharged, Crooke, obtained damages of £100 against Dr Lalor, the Richmond asylum superintendent. It was as a result of this verdict that the inspector of lunatics urged the amendment

of the Irish Lunacy Acts to make the committal order and certificates a justification for confinement.[132] The Lunatic Asylums (Ireland) Act of 1875 provided this amendment for both public and private asylums and also enacted that incorrect or defective certificates could be corrected within fourteen days of the committal.[133]

This amendment to the law effectively placed the ordinary lunatic on the same plane as the dangerous lunatic. An action after this date would rest on lack of jurisdiction, conspiracy, or perhaps the legitimacy of the medical certificate (I am not aware of an Irish case involving this). In 1882 James Coghlan (or Coughlin) sued two magistrates for committing him, and Dr Hatchell (the Maryborough superintendent) for receiving him in the asylum. Following allegations by his solicitor that his committal had been obtained illegally, the inspector and the government legal officers had investigated the case, agreed the committal was irregular and discharged Coghlan. The warrant of committal had not shown the circumstances of his removal to another petty sessions district and the court ruled that the magistrates in committing and the superintendent in receiving him were culpable.[134] Allegations of conspiracy were harder to prove and less successful.[135]

Outside an action by or on behalf of a confined person we may note that the Lord Chancellor could initiate inquiries and set a person at liberty if he thought fit. In such a case in 1892, Lord Ashbourne explained that both he and the registrar in lunacy (an officer responsible to the Lord Chancellor) often went through asylums to see ordinary as well as chancery lunatics; on a visit to the Retreat Asylum in Armagh the registrar had talked to Mrs Martha Godfrey and subsequently referred her case to the Lord Chancellor for investigation. She was found sane and Lord Ashbourne directed that she be allowed to choose where she wanted to go, as there was some friction between herself (a Catholic convert) and her family (who were Protestant).[136]

The 'paternal character' of lunacy law and its practice may be seen as deriving from the medieval prerogative jurisdiction over lunatics and idiots. But developments in the nineteenth century had substantially altered the relation between the lunatic and society. Where the royal prerogative had been exercised (and was, of course, still exercised in the nineteenth century) for the protection of lunatics, or more particularly their estates, the new jurisdiction over lunatics in the shape of 'dangerous lunatic' and lunatic asylum statutes was exercised as much for the protection of society as for that of the lunatic. While, for example, the position of the Lord Chancellor in relation to

chancery lunatics was virtually to speak on behalf of the person confined, the law did nothing to provide a spokesman for the lunatic in 'ordinary' or 'dangerous' committals. An institutional protection, in the shape of the inspectorate, was established; but, as the chief justice in the Dublin case *Re Crooke* [1870] noted, the inspector of lunatics, Dr Nugent, had informed him that he had 8,000 lunatics under his charge and it was impossible to give personal attention to each case.[137] And even where money, an interested friend or the initiative of the confined person brought a case to court, past illegalities could be excused by the present condition of the alleged lunatic. In this way the institutional solution to a problem of social order, even where it exceeded the bounds of law in the first place, could be rationalised as legitimate by the courts at a later date. The social necessity of restraining the dangerous was seen to overrule questions of individual liberty long before turn-of-the-century reformers began to put forward their collectivist programmes for the restraint of degenerates.

In terms of their impact on society at large, the nineteenth-century laws for the confinement of lunatics were of much greater significance than the innovations in the law regarding criminal responsibility of the insane, on which so much has been written. The former registrar in lunacy in Ireland, whose chief business was the administration of the law regarding chancery lunatics, considered the law relating to lunatic asylums needed little commentary. It was, he said,

> one of the great merits of the code that it works in a smooth routine, and is generally so well administered and well understood as to leave comparatively small room for the emerging of legal difficulties.[138]

Certainly, as we have seen, few legal difficulties did emerge, at least in Ireland. The questions thrown up by the laws of certification and confinement were primarily social and ethical. They concerned the administration and control of the lives of those deemed insane by the sane, magistrates, police, doctors and not least, relatives or friends. The last group were probably the most important in determining who the insane were, and their importance will be examined in the next chapter. By making possible the expeditious confinement of an offending family member, the law played a major role in recasting relationships of violence or incompatibility into an opposition of sane and insane individuals.

Notes

1. The history of developments in this area in England is covered in N. Walker, *Crime and Insanity in England Volume One: The Historical Perspective* (University Press, Edinburgh, 1968).

2. Cf. P. McCandless, 'Liberty and Lunacy: The Victorians and Wrongful Confinement', *Journal of Social History*, vol. 11, no. 3 (1978), pp. 366-86.

3. 12 Anne (II), c. 23 and 17 Geo. II, c. 5; cf. K. Jones, *A History of the Mental Health Services* (Routledge, London, 1972), pp. 25-8 and W.Ll. Parry-Jones, *The Trade in Lunacy* (Routledge, London, 1972), p. 7.

4. Cf. 17 Geo. II, c. 5, s. 20 referring to 'the reasonable Charges of removing and of keeping, maintaining, and curing such Person during such Restraint'.

5. See Parry-Jones, *Trade in Lunacy*, pp. 13-14.

6. Walker, *Crime and Insanity in England*, pp. 66-72.

7. 39 & 40 Geo. III, c. 94, s. 3.

8. *Select Committee on Criminal and Pauper Lunatics*, p. 11, *HC* (1807), ii. The report of the committee (p. 4) says that only 37 lunatics had been proceeded against under the 40 Geo. III but this refers probably to criminal lunatics only (i.e. under section 1).

9. On Paul, see R.A. Cooper, 'Ideas and their Execution: English Prison Reform', *Eighteenth Century Studies*, vol. 10 (1976-7), pp. 73-93, and the 1807 select committee (note 8), pp. 14-21. On the rationale of separating lunatics from prisoners, see Scull, *Museums of Madness: The Social Organization of Insanity in Nineteenth-Century England* (Allen Lane, London, 1969), pp. 40-2.

10. 1 & 2 Vic., c. 14, s. 2.

11. 1 & 2 Geo. IV, c. 33, ss. 16-18.

12. *8th Report*, p. 28, *HC* (1857), sess. II, xvii.

13. 1 Vic., c. 27, s. 1; the remainder of the Act dealt with criminals who became lunatic in gaol and could be transferred to asylums.

14. See Chapter 1.

15. 5 & 6 Vic., c. 123, ss. 14, 15.

16. *Report from the Select Committee ... to consider the state of the Lunatic Poor in Ireland*, pp. viii, xxv, *HC* (1843), x; *Correspondence between the Irish Government and the Managers of District Lunatic Asylums, HC* (1844), xliii.

17. For the inspectors' report of 1847 and subsequent correspondence dealing with these administrative changes, see *Report*, Appendix, pp. 19-23, *HC* (1849), xxiii.

18. *Royal Commission*, Appendix, p. 89, *HC* (1857-8), x.

19. *8th Report*, p. 16, *HC* (1857), sess. II, xvii.

20. RP 1861/6868.

21. *8th Report*, p. 81, *HC* (1857), sess. II, xvii; *11th Report*, p. 25, *HC* (1862), xxiii.

22. *Royal Commission*, ev. 3798-3800, *HC* (1857-8), xxvii.

23. *9th Report*, p. 459, *HC* (1859), sess. II, x; *13th Report*, p. 52, *HC* (1864), xxiii; *11th Report*, p. 25, *HC* (1862), xxiii; *13th Report*, p. 50.

24. *Hansard*, 3rd ser., vol. 68, 885-7 (25 April 1843).

25. *Hansard*, 3rd ser., vol. 179, 591 (31 March 1865) (E. McEvoy, MP for Meath).

26. *Select Committee*, pp. xii-xiv, *HC* (1843), x.

27. *Royal Commission*, p. 21, *HC* (1857-8), xxvii.

28. *Hansard*, 3rd ser., vol. 179, 591 (31 March 1865), and ibid., vol. 170, 989 (30 April 1863).

29. *14th Report*, p. 20, *HC* (1865), xxi; also *9th Report*, p. 17, *HC* (1859), sess. II, x for similar objections.

30. In the two years and nine months to 31 December 1862, 31·8 per cent of male and 22·7 per cent of female admissions to district asylums were 'dangerous lunatics'

committed on the viceregal warranty; had all those committed to gaol been sent direct to asylums the proportion of male and female 'dangerous lunatics' to total admissions would have been 49·8 per cent and 34·7 per cent respectively.

31. *Hansard*, 3rd ser., vol. 188, 1314-16 (9 July 1867).

32. 30 & 31 Vic., c. 118, s. 10.

33. RP 1876/19445.

34. RP 1868/13814. As in England, workhouses in Ireland were used for the maintenance of some pauper lunatics but not so much as a matter of policy as through default of asylum capacity.

35. RP 1868/13814.

36. RP 1876/19445.

37. RP 1869/14589.

38. RP 1868/7733.

39. *18th Report*, p. 14, *HC* (1868-9), xxvii.

40. Ibid., pp. 5-6.

41. This was a rosy view of previous magisterial practice and contradicted the inspectors' own judgement of only a year before that under the old Act (1 Vic., c. 27 and 8 & 9 Vic., c. 107):

> parties bringing lunatics before Justices have found no difficulty in deposing to facts sufficient to give a colour to the case even though the individuals might be perfectly harmless, and thus secure their committal as dangerous.

17th Report, p. 31, *HC* (1867-8), xxxi.

42. *18th Report*, p. 8, *HC* (1868-9), xxvii.

43. RP 1872/16659, 1883/19710; cf. RP 1879/19520, for a similar case in Mayo.

44. *19th Report*, p. 6, *HC* (1870), xxxi.

45. RP 1899/20609.

46. 38 & 39 Vic., c. 67, s. 5.

47. RP 1894/12452, 1888/3327, 1904/4269.

48. RP 1876/17934 (1875 circular); RP 1894/12452 (1883); *MPC* Irish Supplement, 22 June 1892 (1892); RP 1895/11256 (1895).

49. RP 1897/16840.

50. Cf. *43rd Report*, p. 2, *HC* (1894), xliii, where the inspectors claim that relatives are unwilling to use the 'dangerous lunatic' procedure in the case of females. Drunken persons, of course, could be taken into custody by the police; once arrested they would usually be prosecuted as drunken and disorderly under the Licensing Acts. In 1881 for instance 68,056 males and 10,517 females were prosecuted in this way (*Judicial statistics for Ireland* (1881), p. 94, *HC* (1882), lxxv). Inevitably the police decided that some of this great number might be suitable cases for asylum treatment. The contribution of drunkenness to asylum populations was a matter of debate throughout the period covered by this book so any estimates of 'drink as a cause of committal' are clouded by various forms of bias. However, the evidence of a balanced and respected observer, Conolly Norman (superintendent of the Richmond asylum), was that alcoholism was a 'chief cause' of admission in about one-third of male admissions from 1901 to 1904 but in less than one-fifth of female cases in the same period. See his evidence to the *Royal Commission on the Care and Control of the Feeble-Minded*, ev. 22836, *HC* (1908), xxxvii. For drink as a cause of committal, see below, pp. 146-50.

51. *MPC*, 16 March 1881, 14 September 1881.

52. *Report of the Commissioners appointed to inquire (inter alia) whether any additional and other provision is required for the better care, relief, and treatment of the poor who are lunatic, idiotic and imbecile in mind ...*, (Trench Commission hereafter), Appendix, p. 230, *HC* (1878-9), xxxi.

53. *Mitchell Committee*, 2nd report, p. 34, *HC* (1890-1), xxxvi.

54. *Trench Commission*, ev. 1609-19, *HC* (1878-9), xxxi.

55. Among his many other posts, William Neilson Hancock (1820-88) had acted as Clerk of Papers in matters of idiots and lunatics in the Irish Court of Chancery from 1855-8 and 1859-60. For a brief profile see R.D.C. Black, *The Statistical and Social Inquiry Society of Ireland Centenary Volume 1847-1947* (Dublin, 1947), pp. 57-61; see the society's *Journal* (hereafter *SSISI*), vol. 6 (1871-6), p. 502, for the formation of a Charity Organisation Committee in December 1875; ibid., vol. 7 (1876-9), pp. 136-7 for the committee's report on 'imbeciles, idiots and harmless lunatics'; ibid., vol. 7, pp. 6-8 for a call for assimilation of the Irish law to English (by John Lentaigne, president in 1877) and ibid., vol. 8 (1880-4), pp. 79-82 for a similar call by Hancock in 1879.

56. Ibid., vol. 8, pp. 316ff. for O'Hagan's presidential address to the Social Science Congress in Dublin 1881.

57. RP 1883/17018 for opposition to the Bill. Although most protests related to the change in the taxation base (from the county cess to the poor rate) for care of lunatics the Mayo grand jurors delivered an unusual critique of the Bill's purpose:

> We think it is wrong and impolitic to give Police and Relieving Officers a pecuniary interest in the arrest and detention of a poor, harmless and unprotected class of people; and we cannot doubt that the effect of such a measure would be to cause much misery and unhappiness to people whose life, on the whole may be as enjoyable to themselves as that of others more intellectually gifted.

See *Hansard*, 3rd ser., vol. 277, 940-1 (20 March 1883); vol. 280, 780 (18 June 1883); vol. 281, 178 (3 July 1883) for the Bill in Parliament.

58. RP 1876/19445, enclosing 1876/15913.

59. For the inspectors' advocacy of amendment in the 1890s and 1900s see RP 1906/2070 (their report of 1893 on defects in lunacy administration) and RP 1907/12449; for the medical profession, see *MPC*, 16 May 1888 (criticism of the Irish admissions system at the British Medical Association Congress in 1888) and RP 1907/12449 (the amendments proposed by the Medico-Psychological Association); see also *Mitchell Committee*, pp. 33-42, *HC* (1890-1), 36, which criticised the Irish lunacy law on the grounds that it was an order of indefinite detention, making no provision for review of the detainee's status (unlike the revised English lunacy law of 1890).

60. G.W. Abraham, *The Law and Practice of Lunacy in Ireland* (Dublin, 1886), p. 431.

61. The situation in Ireland in the nineteenth century was much the same as in the United States today where the great majority of committals to mental hospitals are compulsory. Cf. Saleem A. Shah, 'Dangerousness and Civil Commitment of the Mentally Ill: Some Public Policy Considerations', *American Journal of Psychiatry*, vol. 132 (1975), pp. 501-5, which points out that the 'mentally ill' population is at least not any more dangerous than a number of other groups in the community who are not subject to compulsory detention; and that psychiatry is unable to predict dangerousness anyway.

62. For the background to the formation of the constabulary see G. Broeker, *Rural Disorder and Police Reform in Ireland, 1812-36* (Routledge and Kegan Paul, London, 1970) and K. Boyle, 'Police in Ireland before the Union', *Irish Jurist* (n. s.), vol. vii (1972), pp. 115-35.

63. From a letter cited in *SSISI*, vol. 2 (1857-60), p. 429.

64. RP 1844/A17206, 1888/5486, 1893/8613, 1902/16946, 1903/10397.

65. RP 1871/21394.

66. RP 1854/19057.

67. *The Royal Irish Constabulary Manual; or Guide to the Discharge of Police Duties* (Dublin, 1898) (1st edn 1866), p. 19.

68. RP 1907/28750.

69. Cf. RP 1897/18168, 1898/10170.

70. RP 1897/5767.

71. RP 1845/G8338, G2338; cf. RP 1877/827 for a similar directive to the police to watch an individual closely in order that he be arrested for a crime to which he might plead insanity.

72. RP 1894/12913, 1909/22281.

73. 38 & 39 Vic., c. 67, ss. 3, 4.

74. RP 1879/8412.

75. RP 1890/764.

76. It was not only a tiresome but a frustrating business. Margaret P. was committed at Nenagh at 3.40 p.m. on 24 October 1872. The Bridewell keeper refused to keep her overnight so the police took her direct to Clonmel, arriving at 4.00 a.m. the following morning after a journey of over 50 miles. The gate-keeper told them no cases were admitted until after 9.00 a.m. and went away, leaving them in heavy rain and a strong wind until 6.15 a.m. when he returned and received the patient—the final ignominy for the police was being handed a receipt for the woman, marked '4.00 a.m.' RP 1876/17934 (encl. 1872/17956).

77. Andrew Reed, *The Irish Constable's Guide* ... (Dublin, 1880), pp. 171-2.

78. RP 1876/17934.

79. RP 1876/5756.

80. Richmond Lunatic Asylum, Male Case Books (1905-6) p. 145 (hereafter RMCB).

81. For the violence involved prior to the committal, see below, pp. 155-6, also RP 1875/16179, 1876/17934.

82. R.J. Kinkead, *The Guide for Irish Medical Practitioners* (Dublin, 1889), p. 155.

83. 14 & 15 Vic., c. 68, s. 15; cf. *MPC*, Irish Supplement, 10 January 1877.

84. *MPC*, 19 September 1849. In Dublin, the police magistrates were paid out of a trial fund. The law did not specify that a doctor should be paid and it is evident from this reference that there was pressure on him to attend gratuitously.

85. 38 & 39 Vic., c. 67, s. 14. An attempt had been made to introduce a lunacy fee in 1871, RP 1871/14191.

86. Kinkead, *Guide for Irish Medical Practitioners*, p. 156; *MPC*, Irish Supplement, 12 June 1878 and 25 June 1884 where the granting of fees is listed as one of the major achievements of the IMA amounting to about £1,600 per annum to the profession in Ireland.

87. *MPC*, 6 November 1878; cf. *MPC*, 12 August 1885.

88. *Irish Law Times and Solicitor's Journal*, 4 October 1884.

89. RP 1860/12232.

90. HOS 29/1/5/5231, Public Record Office of Northern Ireland (PRONI).

91. RP 1872/3654.

92. HOS 29/1/5/5248, PRONI.

93. *Royal Commission*, ev. 3746-84, *HC* (1857-8), xxvii.

94. *MPC*, 20 December 1905.

95. *Royal Commission on the Poor Laws*, Appendix to the tenth volume of evidence, p. 110, *HC* (1910), l.

96. Thus in the year ended 30 September 1890, one medical officer in the Monaghan dispensary district certified 19 people; in a similarly sized district (Clonakilty, Co. Cork) none were certified. *Nineteenth Annual Report of the Local Government Board (Ireland)*, Appendix E *HC* (1890-1), xxxv.

97. RP 1906/12636; *MPC*, Irish Supplement, 4 September 1895—'The examination of lunatics is, according to law, entrusted not to the doctor who is conversant with the case, but to a practitioner who happens to reside in the petty sessions town, who has no knowledge of the circumstances.'

98. RP 1898/10170, 1909/3902; *MPC*, Irish Supplement, 11 June 1879.

99. Cf. *MPC*, Irish Supplement, 20 November 1878, ibid., 6 June 1883. The Irish

supplement of the *Medical Press and Circular* includes numerous examples of two pounds or two guineas being charged for lunacy committals. The Mountmellick guardians regarded a 'reasonable fee' for this as the usual doctor's fee of one guinea, *MPC*, Irish Supplement, 25 November 1879.

100. *MPC*, Irish Supplement, 13 June 1877, 10 April 1878, 17 February 1909.

101. *MPC*, Irish Supplement, 9 July 1879 and 25 September 1879 for one such case and the guardians' reactions. Cf. Kinkead, *Guide for Irish Medical Practitioners*, p. 157. For later attempts to control the level of fees see *MPC*, Irish Supplement, 6 January 1892 (Tullamore), 5 June 1895 (Granard) and 23 September 1903 (Kilrush).

102. *MPC* Irish Supplement, 28 November 1906 for decision in *Dr King* v. *Delvin Guardians*. After this High Court judgement against the doctors, the courts sometimes reduced the level of fees ordered by justices, *MPC*, Irish Supplement, 28 July 1909 and 17 January 1912.

103. See above, p. 98.

104. *MPC*, Irish Supplement, 24 November 1875.

105. RP 1901/21073.

106. RP 1894/8199—the words used by a magistrate to explain why two private practitioners had been called in to certify a man whom a dispensary doctor had refused to certify.

107. *JMS*, vol. 26 (1880), p. 549, in his reply to the toast at the annual general meeting of the Medico-Psychological Association, July 1880; see also *MPC*, 11 August 1880 for same.

108. See his pamphlet on mentally defective children, enclosed by the Irish division of the NSPCC in a letter urging the government to extend mental deficiency legislation to Ireland, RP 1919/25489.

109. R.J. Sharpe, *The Law of Habeas Corpus* (Clarendon Press, Oxford, 1976), p. 154. The *parens patriae* power derives from the medieval concept of the king's paternal jurisdiction over his subjects, for example in the case of lunatics and idiots. More recently, of course, this power has been vested in the state and used to justify the involuntary detention of the mentally ill for their own good. There is a distinction between this type of state control of the mentally ill and the use of police power, as in the Dangerous Lunatic Acts, which is directed towards protecting the public at large. In practice, however, as recent American critiques have pointed out, police powers are frequently invoked for *parens patriae* purposes. This was certainly the case in nineteenth-century Ireland. For a discussion of these issues in the American context see Bruce J. Ennis and Richard D. Emery, *The Rights of Mental Patients* (Avon Books, New York, 1978), pp. 35-52 and Nicholas N. Kittrie, *The Right To be Different* (Pelican, Harmondsworth, 1973), ch. 1.

110. 1 & 2 Vic., c. 27, s. 2.

111. 8 & 9 Vic., c. 107, s. 11.

112. 9 & 10 Vic., c. 115, s. 3.

113. 30 & 31 Vic., c. 118, s. 11.

114. RP 1862/13259.

115. RP 1870/15398.

116. RP 1899/23778.

117. *Re O'Reilly* (1894), 29 *Irish Law Times Reports* 33.

118. RP 1874/6284.

119. RP 1879/19839.

120. 5 & 6 Vic., c. 123, ss. 27-9, 38; 8 & 9 Vic., c. 107, ss. 23-4.

121. RP 1847/G6223.

122. RP 1878/10404.

123. RP 1853/7870.

124. RP 1892/16168.

125. RP 1860/12232.

126. Sharpe, *Law of Habeas Corpus*, pp. 152-3. Cf. In *Re Philip Clarke* [1950]

Irish Reports 235 where the judge discharged a habeas corpus application and described the Mental Treatment Act of 1945 as of a 'paternal character', not infringing the rights of the citizen under the Irish constitution: J.M. Kelly, *Fundamental Rights in the Irish Law and Constitution* (2nd edn) (Allen Figgis, Dublin, 1967), p. 97.

127. *R.* v. *Riall* (1860), 11 *Irish Common Law Reports* 279.

128. *Re O'Reilly* (note 117 above); the English cases were *Re Shuttleworth* [1846] 9 QB 651 and *R.* v. *Pinder, Re Greenwood* [1855] 24 LJ QB 148, cf. Sharpe, *Law of Habeas Corpus*, p. 152.

129. *MPC*, 30 December 1868. I have not been able to locate the source of this case, possibly heard in England.

130. Sharpe, *Law of Habeas Corpus*, p. 153. Following one such case in England in 1956, some 3,000 other patients who had been improperly committed were discharged.

131. RP 1879/6200.

132. RP 1874/7951 and 1875/13462 (ending 1875/1566) for details of the case and subsequent correspondence on the state of the law in Ireland; cf. also *MPC*, 21 June 1871.

133. 38 & 39 Vic., c. 67, ss. 3-5.

134. *Coghlan* v. *Woods, Molloy and Hatchell* [1882] 10 *Irish Law Reports* 29 and 16 *Irish Law Times Reports*, 105; RP 1881/20042.

135. *Hutchinson* v. *Walsh and another* (1904) 38 *Irish Law Times Reports* 133; also RP 1907/10247 for another case.

136. *Re Godfrey* (1892), 29 *Irish Law Times Reports* 278.

137. See report of case in *Daily Express*, 11 May 1870, (press cutting in RP 1874/7951). Since Irish lunacy law remained unreformed until well into this century there was no routine review of a patient's status. In 1903 Conolly Norman of the Richmond asylum regretted the absence of the English requirement that a patient be recertified every year. *JMS*, vol. 49 (1903), p. 52.

138. Abraham, *Law and Practice of Lunacy in Ireland*, p. 428.

4 INSANITY: THE CONTEXTS OF COMMITTAL

By the early years of this century, committing a lunatic to the asylum had become a common enough feature of Irish life. The sane, those committing the lunatic, could see this as a violent or distasteful process. On the other hand, it might also be viewed with complaisance by those who had frequently seen the law in action.

The former experience, for instance, is conveyed in a chapter of Sean O'Casey's autobiography. There Cassidy (O'Casey's pseudonym) is forced to arrange the committal to the asylum of his brother-in-law, afflicted with general paralysis of the insane. The context of the man's committal is necessarily violent; Cassidy has to use the leg of a chair to subdue Benson who has once again battered his wife. The time has finally arrived when Benson must be taken off to the 'House of the Dead', the Grangegorman (Richmond) asylum in Dublin. Sean Cassidy's brief visit to the asylum is conveyed with a gothic horror at this institution which houses a bizarre collection of patients, keepers and doctors. The asylum presents a fearful face. Committal there arises in a context of ugliness and degrading brutality.[1]

A different impression is gained from a sketch by J.M. Synge. Among the peasants of the Wicklow hills, of Ireland in general, he suggested, the madhouse was less dreaded than the union workhouse. The union, a home of refuge for 'tramps and tinkers', was looked on with supreme horror by the peasants; the asylum they knew better. Certainly, as we have already suggested, the workhouse was a much less significant institution after the 1850s. Contrariwise the asylum's importance had grown from decade to decade. Indeed by the 1900s the problem of peasant society, on Synge's account, is no longer destitution but rather the fracturing of the old society. He identifies life in the hills of Wicklow with a tendency to 'nervous depression', springing variously from the climate and atmosphere of the mountains to the isolation arising from the breakdown of traditional society.[2] In such a context, he seems to suggest, the asylum has a function more benign than suggested by O'Casey's picture of violence and despair. In the one account, the committal derives from the necessity of self-defence, from the interests of the sane; in the other, from the need to provide refuge for the insane. In this chapter we want to outline the social contexts of committal in order to evaluate the relative

significance of these two functions of the asylum. But first, just how common had committal become by 1900?

Demographic and Social Features

In 1851 some 950 people had been admitted to the public asylums. At a time when the workhouses still held nearly 170,000 paupers there were little more than 3,000 asylum inmates. At just 14·5 admissions per 100,000 population the 'lunacy rate' was not startling. Half a century later the difference was remarkable. With over 2,800 *first* admissions in 1901, increasing to well over 3,000 in the following few years, the lunacy figures were making some asylum authorities and doctors anxious. The actual numbers admitted had tripled; but during a half-century of population decline the admission rate had grown more than four-fold to 63·4 per 100,000. Compared to the workhouse the social significance of the asylum had increased dramatically. By 1906, when a census of paupers in Ireland was conducted, there were just over 36,000 in workhouses (40,000 were on outdoor relief). Synge's impression that the asylum was better known to the Irish peasantry than the workhouse gains statistical substance from the age-distribution of each institution's population. If we exclude the lunatic and idiot inmates (some 8 per cent of the workhouse population in 1906) the majority of workhouse inmates were over 60 years of age.[3] The workhouse had become primarily a geriatric institution. Indeed the poor relief system as a whole (for the overwhelming majority of outdoor relief was paid to those over 60) was an institution for the support of people who had passed their productive years and were increasingly left destitute by, for instance, the emigration of children or relatives who once might have supported them in old age. The asylum, on the other hand, most frequently admitted people in the early and middle stages of their adult life. By the early 1900s even the asylum's permanent population (which was somewhat older than those admitted from year to year) was still quite young. In 1901 only one in seven inmates was aged over 60 years.[4]

The relatively youthful nature of the asylum population had always been evident. As the age-specific admission rates (Table 2) demonstrate, from 1861 to 1901 all age-groups, of both sexes, showed dramatic increases. Of course, there were variations in the rate of this increase. The greatest increment was among the older age-groups, particularly those over 70 years old. And women almost invariably were less vulnerable to committal than men. Still, the most striking thing about

Table 2: Age-Specific Rates of Admission to District Lunatic Asylums per 100,000

Male	1861	1871	1881	1891	1901
0-9	1·0	0·1	0·3	0·6	0·4
10-19	10·7	14·2	18·3	22·6	25·7
20-29	42·2	95·8	101·3	131·5	156·3
30-39	46·9	107·8	122·7	157·8	180·0
40-49	31·2	81·1	98·0	128·7	150·5
50-59	26·7	59·0	69·6	105·6	128·3
60-69	19·7	47·4	56·8	79·5	105·8
70+	5·8	25·2	33·0	49·9	75·1
Female					
0-9	0·7	0·1	0·1	—	0·2
10-19	12·1	15·6	14·6	19·6	23·6
20-29	34·0	68·9	78·2	95·3	109·4
30-39	45·5	79·9	97·3	125·4	146·6
40-49	35·4	60·7	81·1	113·5	129·6
50-59	36·1	51·7	59·4	87·6	110·3
60-69	18·5	36·2	41·6	63·0	82·6
70+	12·0	18·0	21·2	30·9	59·7

Source: Annual reports of the inspectors of lunatics.

the insane was their youth. For both sexes the most vulnerable period was the 30s, but even in their 20s and 40s both men and women showed consistently high admission rates.

The insane were characterised not only by their relative youth and the preponderance of males but also by their marital status which was more generally single. Again this is not surprising when one considers

Table 3: Marital Status—Percentage of Asylum Admissions (1891, 1901, 1911) and Percentage of Asylum Residents (1871, 1881)

Male	1871	1881	1891	1901	1911
Married	18·3	20·4	28·5	28·0	25·5
Single	74·6	71·8	64·6	65·0	67·0
Widowed	3·3	4·0	3·1	4·0	4·7
Not known	3·8	3·8	3·8	3·1	2·9
Female					
Married	22·2	26·1	33·7	29·5	30·3
Single	63·8	61·0	53·9	58·7	58·7
Widowed	9·8	8·6	9·9	10·1	9·4
Not known	4·1	4·3	2·4	1·7	1·6

Source: Annual reports of the inspectors of lunatics.

the declining marriage rate after the Famine—but it was a matter of some note to English observers who found in this detail a contrast with the English situation where the married were predominant. As Table 3 shows, there were important consequences for the permanence of asylum populations arising from the relative numbers of single and married admitted.

As compared with the general population, the proportion of male admissions who were single in 1901 was some 7 per cent greater; in the case of women, some 9 per cent. The proportion married in the Irish population in 1901 was 37 per cent—the percentage of asylum admissions married was less than 30. Once in the asylum it seems it was less likely that a person would be taken out or released again if he or she was single; for this reason the percentage of single persons resident (as suggested by the figures for 1871 and 1881) was somewhat greater than of those admitted. Inside the asylum the single had, of course, no chance of marrying; if they got out they might bear the stigma of having been committed. And if insanity was predominantly a characteristic of youth (particularly among males) then it is hardly surprising to find such a high proportion of single people in the asylum population at a time when the tendency in Irish society was to delay or even avoid marriage.[5]

Singleness did not necessarily mean *social* isolation, a problem which has been implicated as most serious in twentieth-century studies of rural Irish society.[6] As we will suggest later in this chapter, insanity presented itself most commonly in the nineteenth century in a family context. The nature of the records makes this a difficult matter to substantiate. Of the 160 admissions to the Omagh asylum in 1871 admission warrants survive for 133. From these we can learn that 108 had an immediate relative living in the same locality—the evidence given is rarely sufficient to establish whether they are living in the same house, but this appears to have been the case in most instances. In later years when records are more complete this proportion (over 80 per cent) appears to have been the same. Perhaps there is some significance in the decline of this figure by 1901 to only 74 per cent: even in the Omagh district where emigration had been barely equal to the Irish average (that is much less than in the south or west) its isolating consequences were possibly becoming evident.[7]

The occupational origins of the institutionalised insane are frequently more obscure than their demographic characteristics. Insanity, John Conolly commented in 1858, was a 'great leveller'[8] and one found in the public asylums, of Ireland at least, professional people, clerics,

shopkeepers, independent farmers, in other words, people who were usually ineligible for relief. While the asylums were intended for the 'lunatic poor' there was no accepted definition of this category: there were frequent complaints that asylums were admitting those quite capable of contributing to their support. In most cases such admissions were through the medium of the Dangerous Lunatics Act; but, as the asylum became more respectable, paying patients were more common. Consequently any assessment of the asylum's social character must recognise a rather broader spectrum than the phrase 'asylums for the lunatic poor' implies.

Further, information on occupation is too inadequate to allow more than an impressionistic survey from official statistics. Occupation tables are not available in the later official reports. And the earlier evidence is ambiguous with all-encompassing classifications such as 'labouring class' and 'farming class' covering the bulk of admissions. Confidence in these tables is not increased when one is aware of the slipshod information on which they are sometimes based. The wife of an Antrim 'labourer' on a committal warrant in 1891 becomes the wife of a 'respectable farmer' in a police report on the same file.[9] A young man committed to the Richmond asylum from his home near the centre of Dublin is described as a 'farmer's apprentice', but later as a 'farmer'.[10] In some asylums the largest category is merely 'various employments' (Belfast and Carlow in 1861). Even if more accurate information were available about the insane its significance might be obscured when compared with the census occupation tables which are themselves so amorphous. However, given these shortcomings, the following is the general picture of the social origins of the insane.

Of those resident in district asylums in 1871 nearly 19 per cent were listed as having an unknown or no previous occupation. This status could vary greatly throughout the country, being double that figure in the Richmond (Dublin district) asylum. However, since the latter asylum listed 60 per cent of its female inmates as having no occupation, the variations in this category may be due more to different principles of classification adopted by the medical superintendents than a reflection of regional variations. In particular, there seems to be some confusion in the statistics as to whether married women should be included under their husbands' employment when they have no separate employment. For this reason it will be more instructive to separate male and female occupations.

The inhabitants of the asylums were variously described by the inspectors as from the 'agricultural classes', the 'peasant class', the

'lower classes', the 'humbler classes'. Yet 'as a general rule', they claimed, 'mental affections present no variation in the different grades of life.'[11] In fact, given the social structure of Irish society there is little to surprise us in the social background of the insane. The greatest contribution came from the 'labouring class', in this case usually signifying agricultural labourers. In 1871 nearly 38 per cent of the men and 18 per cent of the women were from this background and in 1881, over 40 per cent and 18 per cent respectively. Overlapping this category in many cases were those of 'farming' occupation who comprised nearly 15 per cent of the men and 11 per cent of the women in 1871 (16·5 per cent and 10·9 per cent in 1881). Aside from these two groups which accounted for over half the asylum population (as indeed they accounted for over half the male working population of Ireland) a number of other occupations stood out. Among women, there were domestic servants (about 20 per cent in both 1871 and 1881) and seamstresses (about 6 per cent in both years)—but these proportions were similar to those in the community at large where, for instance, over 28 per cent of women whose occupations were returned at the 1881 census were in domestic service. The catch-all of 'various employments' accounted for about 7 per cent of both sexes. And of the minor categories we should notice 'clerks', 'carpenters', 'shoemakers' and 'students and teachers', with about 2 per cent (males) each; 'soldiers and military pensioners', 4 per cent; various groups of artisans and tradesmen, as well as police, with about 1 per cent each; with a handful of lawyers, medical men and members of religious communities. Most of these groups did not include women, and the large proportion of women returned with no occupation reflects this. And to remind us of the previous condition of many of the asylum's inhabitants, the tables refer to 'mendicants', 1·5 per cent of the males in 1871 and 1881, and 2·7 and 3·5 per cent of the females respectively.

These figures serve to show the variety of backgrounds of the asylum population. As institutions, however, the asylums were largely moulded by the presence of so many agricultural labourers, in some cases comprising half the asylum population. Hence, the inspectors responded to the charge that Irish asylums were excessively spartan in comparison with the English institutions with the defence that the great proportion of Irish lunatics were agricultural labourers and from 'the humblest walks of life'. Their domestic habits and surroundings did not prepare them to expect any better. The important role given to physical labour as a part of moral treatment

was considered especially appropriate in Ireland. At Mullingar the inspectors hoped there would be up to 100 acres of land attached to the asylum 'particularly as four-fifths of the inmates will consist of the agricultural classes'.[12] Designed for the poor they were; but precisely because of the Dangerous Lunatics Act their population was one which reflected a broader spectrum of Irish society than did the workhouse.

The insane, then, were relatively young, more often single than not, more likely (only by a small degree, however) to be male than female, and predominantly from the peasantry and working class (though probably only to the extent that these classes formed the great majority of Ireland's population anyway). There was one other feature worth remarking. This was the regional variation in admission rates. One study has suggested that before 1900 'there was little

Table 4: First Admission Rates per 10,000 Population to Irish District Asylums, 1871-1911

	1871	1881	1891	1901	1911	Percentage increase 1871-1911
Armagh	2·78	3·32	5·69	5·06	5·19	187
Ballinasloe	2·12	2·78	4·65	5·94	6·35	300
Belfast	2·86	2·99	3·24	5·77	4·73	165
Carlow	3·15	3·28	5·81	5·40	5·06	160
Castlebar	2·49	2·66	5·19	4·86	5·89	237
Clonmel	3·20	3·40	4·81	5·40	5·85	183
Cork	2·99	5·02	4·77	5·89	7·06	308
Derry	3·15	3·45	4·77	5·60	4·94	157
Downpatrick	4·03	3·07	4·36	5·73	4·57	113
Ennis	3·40	3·74	5·35	5·81	6·31	186
Enniscorthy	3·69	3·45	4·90	5·35	6·14	166
Kilkenny	3·32	4·23	4·98	5·85	6·68	201
Killarney	2·86	3·49	5·89	7·60	7·72	270
Letterkenny	3·45	4·48	5·40	6·39	5·40	157
Limerick	4·28	5·35	5·56	6·77	5·40	126
Maryborough	3·86	3·78	5·15	7·01	7·55	196
Monaghan	3·49	3·36	5·64	5·81	7·06	202
Mullingar	3·94	4·94	5·89	6·23	6·77	172
Omagh	4·15	3·82	4·65	6·02	6·06	146
Richmond	5·02	5·81	6·27	7·26	6·52	130
Sligo	2·98	4·03	4·86	7·47	7·80	262
Waterford	4·15	4·94	6·35	7·76	7·22	174

Source: Age and sex standardised rates computed from figures in the annual reports of the inspectors of lunatics and the census of Ireland, 1871-1911.

variation in the regional distribution of Irish first admission rates'.[13] Certainly the striking variations in hospitalisation in Ireland in more recent years (high in the west, falling in the midlands to much lower levels in Dublin) were not as evident in the 1901 figures taken by themselves. Yet if these statistics are looked at over a longer time span it is obvious that a picture of homogeneity for the turn of the century is inadequate. For, as Table 4 shows, in 1871 and for the following two decades admission rates were highest in Dublin and were particularly low in most asylums serving the west: Ballinasloe (Galway and Roscommon), Castlebar (Mayo), Cork, Killarney (Kerry) and Sligo (Sligo and Leitrim). It was these asylums in the west which, by 1911, had doubled or trebled their 1871 admission rates. These regional variations are not wholly explicable in terms of socio-economic change. Clare, Limerick and Donegal already had quite high admission rates in 1871 at a time when their neighbouring western counties were still low. But it would appear that the homogeneity suggested by the 1901 statistics was just one stage in a period of transition which reversed the relative vulnerability of different regions to high hospitalisation. During the period we are examining, use of the asylum increased to a dramatic extent throughout Ireland but particularly so along the western seaboard. To the extent that social structures in the west were progressively fragmented by the two-fold impact of emigration and a decline in marriage the asylum may well have come to absorb some of the casualties of this process. Whether this was one of its functions in the post-Famine period must await more detailed research for particular districts.

These broad demographic and social features tell us something about the insane population, principally from where it was recruited. They do not explain, however, what led such people to be committed. We cannot give a wholly satisfactory account of that process. Nevertheless, we can reconstruct the histories of some of these people to suggest what pattern of behaviour led to an asylum admission and how relatives, companions or strangers reacted to them.

Ill-health

In the first place we should consider the poor physical health of many of those admitted to the asylums. From the earliest inspectorial reports there was evidence of this. It was the more obvious in the poorer areas of Ireland, and during the Famine. Dr Heise of the Ballinasloe asylum reported in 1846 that

the patients have been all of a most wretched class, and chiefly affected with chronic disease ... The destitution and neglect in which they are found to be on their being first brought to the asylum, is frightful in the extreme.[14]

Little had changed in 1914 when the superintendent of Killarney asylum reported that, on medical examination after admission, a small number of the patients were in average health and condition. But

by far the largest number were found to be in a low state of bodily health. This ... was more marked in the case of females, a number of whom looked prematurely aged, and gave a history of having suffered from loss of appetite, constipation, insomnia, and other nervous phenomena for many months before the complete mental breakdown supervened.[15]

The poor health of asylum admissions is difficult to quantify. Some mortality figures for asylums are available from later in the period we are considering. From these it appears that about one in fifty males died within a month of admission and more than this among women. In 1901 and 1911 over 3 per cent of females died within one month of admission and almost another 3 per cent within three months. In the five years, 1889 to 1893, while the majority of asylum deaths occurred among those aged over 45, nearly 30 per cent were among those under 35, that is effectively for the age-group 15 to 35, there being few admissions of children. The major cause of death in the asylum, and the reason for the high mortality of the younger age-groups, was phthisis, or tuberculosis of the lungs. Over 25 per cent of all asylum deaths in 1901 and 1911 were attributed to it, the average age at death being 37 and 39 in these two years. However, while the proportion of deaths in the asylum from tuberculosis probably exceeded the national rate (which was 12 per cent in the decade 1911-20) there was nothing unusual about its impact on the insane; it was also the most important single cause of death outside the asylum. In spite of this, for many years doctors and other observers postulated a nexus between insanity and 'consumption'. No doubt, in the cities, particularly in Dublin, the evidence for this must have appeared overwhelming. The behavioural peculiarities which could accompany advanced tuberculosis were thought by some to constitute a particular type of insanity. Yet with more knowledge of the disease and a close examination of asylum statistics, by about 1900 superintendents feared that their institutions were in fact propagating the disease.[16]

There were other cases in which physical illness and its symptoms were the occasion for admission to the asylum. In hindsight the most obvious example is general paralysis of the insane; its association with earlier syphilitic infection was known only after the turn of the century. While this was a common cause of asylum committal in Britain it was much rarer in Ireland. Indeed, as one Irish doctor with experience in both England and Ireland observed, it was almost unknown in rural Ireland, though more prevalent in Dublin.[17] Aside from this special instance, however, the mental symptoms and intractability of other physically ill people could be cause for committal, among those afflicted with various types of fever, for example. Similarly vulnerable were the aged, whose senility, incontinence or mere ill-temper frequently provoked workhouse officials into sending them to the local asylum. And of course the idiotic, whose condition was not the legitimate object of asylum care, also found their way to these institutions. Such examples illustrate the inadequacy of legal and institutional structures and occasionally the consequences of ignorance or incompetence on the part of medical men, magistrates and police.

Whether a person's behaviour was the result of an insanity or a fever was considered problematical. A local government board inspector was sent to Cork in 1892 to investigate allegations by a parish priest that a dispensary doctor had admitted a lunatic member of a 'fever-stricken family' to a fever hospital, with her mother and sister. Asked why he had done so, the doctor replied:

> because she was a lunatic and because it was an act of charity to do it; besides, it occurred to him that she might have a touch of fever. In assisting to get her removed she became violent and bit him in both hands. At the police barracks he reported his belief that she was a lunatic and gave sworn information to that effect.

The *Medical Press* saw this as an example of the 'difficulties of diagnosis between lunacy and fever delirium well known in general practice and asylums', and drew attention to the 'perplexities of the medical practitioner among the poor and destitute in such cases'.[18] Similarly a 'Practitioner of 40 years' argued that poor diagnosis was leading to the confinement and death in asylums of people who were actually suffering from various diseases such as some forms of meningitis and 'brain fever'.[19] Certainly, in cases of puerperal fever, frequently taken to be puerperal mania and thus reason for committal

to an asylum, the state of a woman's health might be completely ignored.

In 1891 a woman from Larne, near Belfast, was committed on the information of her husband that she had been astray in her mind for three weeks, threatening to kill herself and assaulting him. Although the dispensary doctor certified that she had puerperal fever and 'phlegmasia dolens' (milk-leg or thrombosis), the police were instructed by the magistrates to take her by 'car' to Belfast. On the way she became ill and died while the police were carrying her into a public house. An inspector of lunatics criticised the police for moving her without a medical opinion as to her fitness to travel. In such a case as this, every agent involved was able to rationalise the action—the doctor claimed that there was no place other than the asylum for her; the police that there was no indication from the doctor that she should not travel; the magistrates that she was too violent to be taken by train. In the inspector's opinion she should not have been moved at all.[20] The criterion for committal was the difficulty of management of the woman rather than her mental state—in the doctor's mind the 'mania' obscured the more serious aspect of her condition, the blood-clot, which the inspector claimed would have been moved by the twenty-mile journey to the asylum.

In 1885 a memorial to the Lord-Lieutenant requested an inquiry into the detention in the Down asylum of a woman with puerperal fever and (in the words of the memorialist) 'the mania that often accompanies it'. The doctor explained the committal—she was prematurely confined in early February 1885 (he does not mention that the child died a day later); he visited her three days later and found that she had not been sleeping and had been very nervous before and since her confinement; on the fifth day she became delirious and was constantly talking and singing, she could only sleep under powerful narcotics and would eat only under pressure. The memorialist, brother of the woman concerned, cited another medical opinion that 'it is a grievous wrong to commit as a lunatic one affected as my sister'. Puerperal fever and mania were well known to the profession and their judgement was 'against subjecting the patient to the treatment provided for Lunatics in the ordinary acceptation of the terms'. In this, and no doubt in many cases, there was no consensus of medical opinion—the decision for committal was taken after the superintendent of the Down asylum was called in as 'an expert' and agreed that she should be committed.[21]

Yet such admissions might take place as much through the default

of other institutions as through medical judgement that they were cases suitable only for an asylum. Thus a 21-year-old woman was sent in a delirious state to the Adelaide Hospital in Dublin one week after the birth of her first child. After a week there the matron discharged her as they had 'no convenience for keeping her there'. She was taken to the Chancery Lane police station where her husband, having been told that she had to go to an asylum for any hope of a cure, swore that she was a dangerous lunatic. This being 1862 (that is before the abolition of committal of lunatics to prison) she had first to be sent to Grangegorman penitentiary where she died soon after—the inquest jury found that her death was from 'puerperal mania', accelerated by her removal from the Adelaide Hospital four days earlier.[22] In 1900 another woman 'became insane' after childbirth and was taken to the Coombe Lying-in Hospital (Dublin) by her husband; being considered an unsuitable case, she was refused admission and taken back home; the next day, having 'severely injured herself', she was taken to the workhouse which also refused to admit her and gave her to the police for committal to the Richmond asylum. Admitted there, she died soon after from 'exhaustion and loss of blood'.[23] It is difficult to establish the frequency of such cases—as a proportion of admissions they must have been of minor significance. Yet they demonstrate the importance of the asylum as a receptacle for those whom workhouse, hospital or prison would not house. In these situations the law was conveniently at hand to absolve certain authorities of their responsibilities and to force the hand of others.

A young inmate of the Carrick-on-Suir workhouse was committed as a dangerous lunatic to Clonmel gaol in 1864 where she died six days later from 'mental and bodily exhaustion'. According to the prison medical officer she had 'appeared in a dying state when committed to gaol on 6th [October]'. The master and doctor of the workhouse claimed that they committed her to gaol as the 'readiest means of getting her into the Lunatic Asylums'. Defensively, the doctor continued that he was not aware of anything 'that warrants the conclusion arrived at by the Medical Officer of the gaol that this woman was in a dying state when admitted under his care—she lived for six days'.[24] Such abuse of the law's intended purpose continued even after its amendment in 1867 prohibiting committal to gaol. The convenience of everyday life ensured that this would be so.

Hence in 1872 the ire of the inspectors was raised by 'an instance of the thoughtless committal of persons as *dangerous* lunatics under a recent statute—sent to Asylums on the eve of death, and utterly

prostrate from debility'. The case they cited, however, was less a 'thoughtless committal' than a belated attempt to obtain adequate medical treatment in the face of the refusal by a workhouse hospital to treat a patient. The Fermoy dispensary medical officer explained that he had visited Bridget Morgan, eighteen years old, six weeks before her death. At first she was not confined in bed, but her mother said she had an 'airy fit', was quite silly and talked foolishly. He found her morose and unco-operative. Her mother told him that she had called him in because the neighbours said she had been seduced and was pregnant—she wanted him to disprove this. With the exception of suppression of menstruation, he found no evidence of pregnancy; he prescribed for her, saw her again a couple of days later, when she was still much the same. Called again about five weeks later, he found

> [s]he was violent, her hands were tied across her chest and she
> shouted, cursed, whistled and used the most obscene language.

She had extensive bedsores from lying on a hard, uneven bed. The father wanted her removed to the asylum as he was 'up all night with her and that if she were not removed he would be dead himself'. The doctor agreed. But before signing the certificate two days later, he tried to have her admitted to the workhouse hospital as he feared she would suffer from the bedsores on the long journey to Cork. The workhouse refused, on the grounds that she was 'insane'. So he signed the certificate for her committal, not seeing any reason why she should not be removed. The magistrates 'examined' her, by looking at her in the police car, and she was taken to Cork asylum, a journey of over four hours. There she died thirty hours later. A poor law inspector sent to investigate the case was diffident about whether she should have been removed. He considered the doctor's actions as partly due to his lack of experience in 'mental disease'.

> The flushed face and powerful voice indicated not bodily strength
> but an unnatural excitement of the nervous system, certain (on its
> subsidence) to be followed by an equivalent depression, which in
> Bridget Morgan's case assisted by a low form of bodily disease was
> sufficient to extinguish life.[25]

Here the asylum was functioning as a hospital, though not, we may be sure, the sort of hospital that asylum superintendents wanted to see.
Not all such cases ended for the worse. A young woman, admitted

to the Castlebar asylum in 1870, was described as physically very debilitated though her intellect was 'clear and unclouded'. She had no previous signs of insanity but her husband said she had caught a fever three weeks before and eventually he had to restrain her with ropes. Consequently her wrists were injured, one being cut in three places by the ropes and covered with ulcers. She was committed under the Dangerous Lunatics Act but discharged six weeks later.[26] In all these examples the criteria of insanity were ambiguous, even obscure. Popular and medical opinion equally saw fever, delirium or indeed any behaviour accompanied by sudden alterations in mental states as an 'attack of insanity' and made use of the asylum for its management. That all the examples we have cited were women would seem to reflect more than coincidence: the health risks attendant on pregnancy and childbirth in particular necessarily left women vulnerable to the exercise of this ambiguity in the definition of insanity's boundaries. Committal of such women was but a reflection of the serious stress, both physical and social, placed on them by these major events in their lives. A young and unmarried domestic servant, admitted to the Richmond asylum following a miscarriage and eclampsia, was likely also to have lost her situation as a result of her pregnancy. Bridget P—, who was committed for threatening to take the life of her twelve-day-old child, was ill with fever and pneumonia for a fortnight after her admission; but her recovery within a few more weeks was in contrast to the experience of other 'puerperal' cases admitted about the same time who were dead within a year.[27]

Thus the asylum's function in this respect was a complex one, a consequence of both institutional convenience and contemporary perceptions of insanity. Two other pathways to the asylum, common enough but again marginal to the institution's *raison d'être*, were old age and idiocy. In both cases the absence of other institutions in a society where traditional forms of support for the dependent were declining determined that the old or the idiotic belonged with the insane in asylums.

Old Age

The admissions of those over 70 years of age increased at a rate greater than that of any other age-group throughout the period we are examining. It is hardly surprising, therefore, to find asylum doctors complaining early this century of the increasing committal of old

people to the asylum. This tendency reflected both the growth in relative size of the aged population in Ireland (the proportion over 65 years was 3·6 per cent in 1851; 6 per cent in 1871; 10 per cent in 1911) and the inadequacy of institutional provisions for the aged. The workhouses, of course, took many; but in turn they attempted to transfer this burden to the asylums. While the South Dublin Union agreed with the Richmond asylum committee's position in 1912 that the workhouse should provide for old people and not send them to the asylum, the North Dublin Union claimed it only sent the 'dangerous lunatics'. But Dr Donelan of Richmond countered that the North Dublin workhouse had committed 19 feeble, aged people in 1911 and that the majority of them died within short periods. Others commented on the 'tendency of children of today to transfer their parents to asylums for senile troubles, which formerly were tended in the homes'.[28]

The evidence for this last assertion is difficult to find. The basis for it was the more obvious presence of the aged in the asylum; but as we have seen this was merely a reflection (slightly amplified) of Ireland's ageing population.

Blame could be more personally and concretely laid on the workhouse authorities. Not insanity, not even senility in some cases, but difficulty of management was frequently the criterion of committal from a workhouse. At the Carlow asylum in 1903 Dr O'Meara refused to admit five of the six cases sent to him by the local workhouse, because they were not insane.[29] Faced with such a refusal the workhouse officials could make use of the Dangerous Lunatics Act. An 84-year-old woman in the Bawnboy workhouse (Co. Cavan) was committed to Monaghan asylum in 1893 for having 'attempted' to kick another inmate. Obviously the law was being manipulated for institutional convenience. The warrant was illegal in any case, since the medical certificate was made out by the workhouse and not a dispensary doctor. Required to state the 'species of insanity', the medical officer first wrote 'idiotic', deleted this and replaced it with a genius of his own—'dementia hereditas'. The only evidence of insanity offered was that 'she gets into violent passions without any apparent cause'.[30] The last phrase suggests the ambiguity of 'insanity'. It was not just difficulty of management and control of behaviour which might constitute the disease—it was equally the absence of causes which were accessible to popular, even medical, understanding. It was precisely the ambiguity of the term which made it so useful for disposing of the troublesome, not least when they were old.

Bridget Glennan was arrested at Kinnatty after committing some minor (unspecified) assault and confined as a dangerous lunatic in the Maryborough asylum. An irregularity in the committal brought the case to government notice. On investigation, Inspector Nugent recommended her discharge. She was

> a garrulous, inoffensive old woman—labouring under senile weakness of intellect—probably a person of a hasty or irritable disposition if contradicted—further this female *never* had been deemed insane ...

One of the committing justices defended his action by describing his encounter with her after she was sent back from the asylum for re-examination.

> I put some questions to this Woman, for instance I asked her, 'Where she had been for the past few weeks', her reply, 'I was in my own house & had my two little boys & my little girl with me', this though she had been in the Asylum at Maryboro' during that time, in reply to another question of mine, 'as to how she came into Town today', she said, 'I walked in with my daughter from Kinnatty', though she had a few hours before come by train from Maryboro & in charge of two Policemen.

Having obtained all this apparently conclusive evidence he wanted to commit her. In this case, however, the dispensary doctor (replacing the workhouse doctor in the first examination) considered that she was *not* a lunatic and she was not committed a second time. Yet numerous committals of old people were made in this fashion not because they were dangerous, but because their social dependence in a society faced with an increasing burden of aged left them to the expedient solution of the asylum.[31] Asylum superintendents, for the most part ineffectually, resisted the incursion of the aged, though not always on the ground that they were not insane. Rather, the objection was that such people were incurable and therefore unsuitable to the asylum. As the superintendent of the Ennis asylum described a case sent in from Killadysert workhouse:

> she appears a most unsuitable case for the Asylum being 78 years of age and labouring under senile dementia and I need scarcely remark incurable.

This objection was the more cogent in 1911: the number of aged in asylums swelled the return of incurable cases and 'statistics which included them give a subverted idea of the curative value of asylums'.[32]

Idiocy

The asylum authorities had more success in preventing the admission of the idiotic or mentally retarded. Throughout the century there was a clear distinction between insanity and idiocy. Asylums were intended only for the insane (or lunatic). Nevertheless, among groups whose presence so discomforted the asylum were those described as idiotic or imbecile. Usually the superintendent tried to remove them to the workhouse. Sarah Hogan, described as demented and idiotic as a result of some cerebral disease, was committed to Limerick asylum in 1888. She had been violent for four weeks, assaulting her mother (no details are given) and breaking crockery in the house. The superintendent considered she was a 'wretched imbecile', utterly helpless and not a dangerous lunatic. Her mother was asked if she would send her to the workhouse if she was discharged from the asylum. She agreed to this.[33] In 1872 a Tyrone clergyman wanted the Chief Secretary to make an order committing an idiot boy of seventeen to the asylum. He had already been refused by the Dungannon workhouse because the boy would be a 'troublesome inmate', and by the Omagh asylum because they had no room. The boy was a 'harmless idiot', and one of five children of a labourer, 'but is now become very troublesome & opposes his Mother's authority when his Father is absent'. On advice from an inspector of lunatics, Dublin Castle replied that he should be admitted to the workhouse. Such cases were not for the asylum, the inspector wrote:

> The occupation of beds in asylums by those who with *care* could be fairly treated in poorhouses when quiet is not only *doubly* expenses [*sic*] on rate payers but interferes with the reception of curable or *truly* dangerous cases.[34]

The governors at Castlebar refused to admit an imbecile child of nine years in 1898 because they did not 'consider the Asylum the proper institution for the care and treatment of such a case'.[35] Yet if action was taken under the Dangerous Lunatics Act there was little the

asylums could do. An 'idiotic' child of ten was committed in 1869 to the Cork asylum—how such a child could be considered as dangerous was beyond the inspectors' comprehension, but it was not uncommon.[36] In some cases, however, the asylum superintendent and the inspectors in Dublin challenged such actions. Thus a thirteen-year-old girl in Sligo asylum was discharged after the government law adviser found the warrant did not show her intention of committing a crime.[37] The almost complete absence of facilities for the care and education of 'idiotic' children (there was but one Irish institution, in Dublin, and this for Protestant children)[38] made it inevitable that some would end up in the asylum. Yet through the sort of resistance just described asylum administrators managed to limit their share of this burden. In 1891 there were only 34 children under fifteen years of age in the public asylums; in 1901, 29; in 1911, 61.

Drunkenness

We have seen how the asylum might be used to house persons whose insanity was questioned by medical administrators who had a certain vision of its function as a 'curative' institution. At the same time, to others, in some cases families, in others police or workhouse masters, the asylum was the most obvious, even the only place where irritating, noisy, disturbing people could be sent. Rarely in the examples we presented above was the matter one of containing dangerous behaviour. It could be quite the opposite where drink was involved. The contribution of drink to the asylum population was usually exaggerated by contemporaries—with heredity it shared the blame for the majority of asylum admissions. But it was doubtless 'associated' with a sizeable proportion of admissions. Lists of 'probable causes' of insanity in the annual reports attribute nearly 9 per cent of admissions in 1891 and over 10 per cent in 1901 to 'intemperance in drink'. Some ended in the asylum after a bout of drinking which led to serious violence. Others went in and out with a frequency which illustrates the relatively benign attitude of the asylum authorities; perhaps it also illustrates the unreliability of 'recovery' statistics as any serious indicator of what the asylum was about.

Daniel Clancy, a publican of Dublin, was first committed as a dangerous lunatic to the Richmond asylum in 1869. By late 1876 he had been admitted no less than sixteen times. On all these occasions his state of mind was attributed to drink and after a short time in the

asylum he would recover and be released. During these years his wife applied to the asylum a number of times for his discharge on recovery in spite of his violence to her. By late 1876, however, she was clearly glad to be rid of him. In a petition she complained that he had been released too soon from the asylum. This petition made no mention whatever of his drinking and concentrated instead on his violence—he had tried to cut her throat with a razor whilst she was in bed (the first committal); stabbed himself with a bread knife; and done other unstated violence to herself and their five children. What had happened to change her mind was not clear but a letter written over a year earlier exhibited quite a different tone. There she admits his drinking ('the smallest quantity' affects him 'dreadfully'); the children fret for him; she is afraid that the effect of not being released will permanently impair 'his bodily health'; and although

> [h]is most determined attempts were always at myself ... no matter what affliction he might heap on me I would not wish him to be detained one hour longer than was necessary to restore him to health.

Finally she adds that if he ever be admitted again she will not apply for his discharge. Perhaps her petition of 1876 was merely fulfilling this promise. There is no record of the sequel to these events. However, the law adviser recommended that, since there was little else left to the asylum than to discharge him each time he recovered, a detective should be detailed to watch him closely. Perhaps he would obtain evidence of a crime to which Clancy could plead insanity and so be detained at the pleasure of the Lord-Lieutenant. The success of this ploy would in part depend on medical evidence—Dr Lalor of the Richmond asylum asserted that Clancy was not insane but merely suffered the 'delirium of intoxicating liquors' and was therefore responsible for his actions.[39]

No doubt this was a story familiar enough to police and asylum staff. In 1904 Dr Drapes of the Enniscorthy asylum blamed excessive drunkenness in Wexford for the increase in insanity. He referred particularly to the problem of habitual drunkards returning to the asylum again and again.[40] But since the *insanity* of a drunkard was questionable, his or her state when not drunk rarely justified long detention, even where families or others wanted it. The consequences of drink were indubitably destructive but the protectors of the public health felt limited in what they could do. The failure of inebriate

reformatories and retreats when they were established early this century was symptomatic of the constraints on compulsory detention of drunkards.[41] In such a situation the asylum was an easy last resort.

On his wife's information Michael Lynch, a solicitor's clerk, was committed to Waterford asylum in December 1900. Prior to this he had been writing letters to the constabulary alleging that a police officer had been inducing his wife to commit perjury and have him committed. He had written, he said, several times to Mr Smith (the police officer) 'in connection with boycotting and intimidation to which I am subjected and a murderous assault that was committed on me'. A police report records that he was subject to 'hallucinations' (delusions may be meant) which got worse when he started drinking. He was discharged from the asylum three months later on the application of his wife who said they were moving to Cork. However, a week later he was re-employed by a solicitor. The latter described him to the police as a very hard-working clerk who

> is subject to delusions, and when he takes drink is not accountable for his actions. He has not been drinking to excess since his discharge from the Asylum.

Still his grievances continued—he wrote to his local MP about the conspiracy against him and asking for an inquiry (this was the origin of the file on the matter). By this stage his fears could feed on the reality that he *had* been committed by his wife and the police. On the other hand, his re-employment, and indeed his wife's request for his release, tells us something about the traffic in and out of the asylum and the degree of tolerance shown towards at least some ex-inmates.[42] Elsewhere drunkenness might not be treated so leniently. In 1897 a police constable was dismissed from the service without pension following his continuing drunkenness. A sergeant reported that he was

> showing signs of his mind being deceased [*sic*]. He was speaking last night of soon getting married to the Hon. Lady Mary Cadogan and that he was going to write a love letter to her.

The police medical attendant at Kildare considered that 'a very little liquor would have the effect of upsetting the Constable'. On his dismissal he was sent to the Enniscorthy asylum.[43] Similarly, in 1871 a police constable was dismissed without pension after twenty-six years' service. He had become insane, so the medical officer

considered, by drinking. Detained in the barracks for four months after his discharge, he was eventually removed to Ballinasloe asylum. Despite appeals from his local MP, the inspector-general of constabulary refused to alter the pension decision.[44] In both these cases the committal to an asylum seems only to have taken place after some history of incidents involving drink. In fact the asylum was not used so much for drunkenness *per se* (for which the law in any case had its own penal provisions) as for cases where it substantially disrupted the life of the individual or his relatives.

Another man, admitted to the Enniscorthy asylum in 1896, had a history of six years' intemperance and had been allegedly insane for the last three years. The superintendent reported that he suffered from insanity as a result of 'drink and heredity' (two of his brothers had been in the asylum and one had died there) and was dangerous when the 'brain is excited by alcohol'. He had twice been imprisoned for threatening or assaulting his wife and had so mismanaged his business that he was obliged to assign it to his brother and his wife. Some governors wanted to discharge him. He was a talented and intelligent man, said the superintendent, who could probably convince a judge and jury that he is not insane; but his wife and three witnesses testified before the board of governors that he had been addicted to drink and had threatened her. While the doctor was sympathetic to a discharge he warned of the violent consequences of the man drinking.[45]

At other times drink presented itself less as the origin of personal troubles than as its consequence. It was said of Daniel Bergin, an inmate of the Richmond asylum, that he had been 'unfortunate in business' and consequently became addicted to drink.[46] Perhaps other things besides drink had troubled the mind of James Howard, an old inmate of the Richmond, who recalled his history for a doctor in the 1890s. In September 1868 he had been received in the asylum from Harold's Cross Prison. Some time before this he had been drinking all night at the wake of a friend. He went to work the following day and attended the burial the day after that.

> On the way home he took a bottle of claret in Marlborough Street. When he reached the Quays he suddenly burst away from his friends and running with great rapidity jumped across the wall and into the Liffey.

He knew he was doing wrong, he told the doctor, but he 'could not resist the temptation. He supposes it was the Devil that tempted him.'

A boat hauled him out and he was taken to the police, where he was probably charged with attempted suicide. From there he went to the prison and then to the asylum—presumably, since this account was taken down thirty years later, he ended his life there.[47]

A solicitor's clerk, two policemen, a man in business, a publican whose occupation was a source of never-ending temptation—these few histories touch only the surface of a much greater problem. Late-Victorian reformers wanted to provide special institutions, inebriate asylums, for such people; but the law was not so ready to enforce compulsory treatment of alcoholism as of insanity. In the meantime drink made its own contribution to the lunatic population since it would not be tolerated elsewhere. In 1896 a police medical officer sent a 'harmless lunatic' suffering from delirium tremens to the lunacy ward of a workhouse. The workhouse doctor objected to receiving such a patient but Dr Speedy (the police doctor) argued that nothing else could be done: a case of delirium tremens would not be received in a Dublin hospital and the guardians were responsible for such a person in the lunacy wards.[48]

Mania and Melancholia

Of the many admissions to the asylum the most common were those known in the nineteenth century as 'maniacs' and 'melancholics'. Imprecise as these categories were, one could, from the many texts available, draw up a picture of the typical features of these insanities. However, our concern here is with the social context of insane behaviour and the way it presented itself to contemporaries. We shall examine these confinements for what they reveal about social tolerance and definitions of the insane and, implicitly, about contemporary limits of behaviour. Whether the occasion for committal was an attempted suicide, a vicious or perhaps trivial assault on a relative, or wandering aimlessly about the countryside, the histories we possess frequently illuminate the complex and troubled pattern of these lives and their interaction with their immediate society. Drink, old age or fever could not explain the insanity of those whom the doctors described as maniac or melancholic. For this reason the insane we deal with below were the typical cases, the ones whose behaviour and mentality most bewildered and disturbed the sane. The nature of insanity, despite the attempts of a putatively scientific medicine to explain it, remained inexplicable throughout the nineteenth

century. While the increase of insanity at large was ascribed to 'civilisation' or more commonly, 'heredity', a recurring explanation of its individual manifestation was that it had pleased God or Providence to afflict a person with insanity.[49] For many there seemed no other explanation for the sudden outbursts of temper and violence, or the breakdown and inability to carry on one's life, two typical preludes to asylum admission.

An attempted suicide was taken to be irrefutable evidence of a person's insanity. The suicide rate itself increased in Ireland in the late nineteenth century and peaked in the first decade of this.[50] Although it is not possible from official statistics to quantify attempted suicide it was a common event among those factors leading to confinement in the asylum. An attempt in itself was not necessary; threats to do away with oneself were commonly cited as indicating the need for asylum care. In Dublin, suicide attempts and threats were frequently associated with the River Liffey and the two canals.

We have already met the case of James Howard, who threw himself into the Liffey after drinking a bottle of wine. A 23-year-old unemployed youth admitted to the Richmond asylum in 1888 that he had 'tried to end his miserable life by throwing himself into the Liffey'. Questioned by the doctor after admission he said he was 'lost ... damned ... can't be forgiven'.[51] A pensioned soldier, who had previously been in the Washington asylum, threw himself in the Liffey to escape his persecutors.[52] An epileptic patient had attempted to jump in 'because he had no work'.[53] A 28-year-old mother of one child was admitted in an hysterical state after threatening to throw herself into the Liffey.[54]

With many of these people we know little of what preceded their various threats and attempts. But a 49-year-old woman living in Middle Abbey St, just one block from the river, recalled the major details. Eight days earlier her daughter had died in the Rotunda Hospital while in childbirth. At the wake she did not drink but a week later she had some whiskey and porter. When she asked for more the people in her house would not let her have it so she ran out of the house. The

next thing she remembers was finding herself on the Quay near Grattan Bridge looking into the Liffey & thinking about her son in America.[55]

From this account it is not clear whether she then jumped in, although

she denied having had any suicidal intent. In any case perhaps it was enough to be behaving strangely about the walls of the quays or on the banks of a canal to attract the interest of a policeman or a passer-by.

A young woman, admitted to the Richmond asylum in 1892, had been arrested on the banks of the Grand Canal by a policeman who asked her where she was going; she said she did not know and he then arrested her saying that she wanted to drown herself, 'which I never thought of'. On her own evidence, however, she was in a distracted state of mind. To the doctor she appeared sad and melancholic; but she gave a 'very coherent' account of herself. A few weeks before she had gone out of the house to get milk, leaving two small children in front of the fire. When she came back she found the older one on fire; the child died some days later in Dun's hospital. She could not sleep or eat after this but took a 'few glasses of porter'.

> One night about 11 o'clock I awoke from my sleep as if out of a dream and went along the Canal on the way to the Hospital— forgetting that the child was dead and buried some days.

It was while in this state that the policeman came across her. She was discharged from the asylum nine days later.[56]

Drowning oneself was, of course, only one of the considerable array of methods attempted or threatened by those who became asylum inmates. Jumping from windows, cutting one's throat, hanging, poisoning, shooting—all these were common threats and modes of occasional attempts. Accompanying the attempts went depression, occasionally religious worries and fears. In one case combining both, the person was not even considered a 'lunatic', though the asylum was deemed the appropriate place to send her. Ellen Reilly, a 28-year-old woman who kept house for her two brothers, was committed to Mullingar asylum on the information of one of them that she threatened to take her own life and 'actually crossed the fields with a view of carrying out the threat'—presumably to drown herself. According to a medical report she was 'depressed generally, and states that her soul is lost, and that the Priest is endeavouring in vain to recover her salvation'.[57] Here the committal to the asylum was largely preventive.

In fact very many of the committals of the 'suicidal' were preventive, a response to an outbreak of violent language, threats, attempts—usually foiled by watchful relatives—to get to a window, or a knife. Francis Prichard, a Fermanagh farmer, committed his 25-

year-old son to the Omagh asylum in 1876 following an attack of 'religious insanity' shortly before. He had attempted to drown himself and, as his father put it, 'wanted a knife threatening to put an end to himself'. Evidently the committal was made reluctantly. His father wrote to Dublin Castle six months after the admission requesting his son's discharge, after it had been refused by the superintendent.

> If I thought it would be so difficult to get him out of the Asylum as it is I would not have sent him to it.

The doctor who had signed the medical certificate also reported that the removal to the asylum was made under the belief that Prichard could at any time take his son out under his own charge again.[58]

Attempted suicide, or the threat of it, shared with violent assault (and, more commonly, the threat of this) the ultimate justification for confinement in the asylum; sometimes the two went together. An adolescent girl from Drumgana in Co. Monaghan was committed by her mother following a trying four weeks of conflict. The girl was reported to be restless and insomniac; a month before she had struck her mother a violent blow on the face injuring the sight of her eye; the previous day she had kicked her mother, struck her with a broomstick and threatened to cut her throat while asleep (they shared the bed); as well she had threatened suicide—'By Jesus I'll do away with myself', her mother reported her as saying. She believed her daughter was 'out of her mind'.[59] When a question of assault charges came up (all the above having been sworn before a justice) the police reported that the mother did not want to press a charge of assault, but only have her committed to the asylum. Sending one's own child to the prison was clearly more odious than recourse to the asylum. A similar motivation was evident in the case of a 35-year-old farmer who was detained as a dangerous lunatic in the asylum in 1882 while awaiting appeal against a sentence for assault on his mother. The latter wrote to the Lord-Lieutenant asking for his conviction to be quashed; if he recovered while in the asylum and was sent to prison for the rest of his sentence 'he would never come out alive'. According to medical evidence this farmer had been a heavy drinker, had attempted to kill his mother and several times assaulted his wife.[60]

While an assault on a stranger would no doubt receive less indulgent treatment the case was clearly different where a family was concerned. Catherine Dempsey, wife of a small farmer (also a dealer in flax who was reported to have lost money in his trade) from near

Coleraine (Co. Derry) swore an information against her husband on 8 February 1862—he had assaulted her several times, sometimes with a hatchet or tongs; beat his children with a chain and other weapons; and that day he had severely wounded his daughter with a shovel saying he would 'have a life'. But she must have had second thoughts about proceeding with her action at this stage. He became quieter, although he was reported to have become ill and deranged on 17 March. It was only on 30 May that she proceeded with her action to commit him as a dangerous lunatic.[61] For a family, perhaps wife and children or a dependent parent, the removal of a bread-winner was the price which had to be considered before committing to the asylum. A 76-year-old man, living with a son and daughter on about three-quarters of an acre of land at Pallaskenry, Co. Limerick, had committed his son to the asylum. The latter had worked for some years in the inland revenue before 'his mind became defective and he was ultimately discharged on a pension of £33 per annum'. For the last sixteen years he had lived with his father but

> Latterly his mind appears to have gone altogether wrong he had been threatening to shoot Priests and he purchased a Revolver and 50 or 60 rounds of ammunition which the Police took from him, fearing he might do harm. I swore an information ...

In a letter to the Lord-Lieutenant he complains that he has thus been deprived of his son's support and asks for a proportion of it to 'keep me out of the Workhouse'.[62] There are similar records of others requesting the discharge of a relative, allegedly recovered, claiming that they were their only or principal support.[63]

But memories of violence meant that in other cases there would be little desire to have the bread-winner of the family back. Hearing of the pending release of Patrick Gill from Galway gaol in 1845, his wife swore before a magistrate that his presence would be a danger to his family. She had given information of his verbal and physical violence against her and her daughter five months before—she was not now convinced that his reported recovery was enough.[64] Fears of further violence were occasionally justified by experience. We can point to cases where appalling murders took place after the discharge of a lunatic—James Heslop who ran 'amuck' in Co. Armagh in 1887 killing three people with a bill hook or Thomas Dykes who stabbed his brother to death shortly after discharge from Cork asylum in 1873.[65] Such events usually encouraged the rigidity of discharge practice. But

even less dramatic happenings demonstrate the fear of violence which could provoke the use of the asylum. George McClean, admitted to the Omagh asylum with 'simple mania' in 1858, was taken out on trial by his wife some months later because McClean's brother had been 'attributing improper motives to her keeping him in the asylum'. After only eight days out he was re-admitted after continual threats to her culminating in him stabbing her in the breast. In the asylum he was again violent but improved so much that his wife took him out again. Still, the resident physician reported, 'she was apprehensive of his doing her some harm'.[66]

The violence which characterised the histories of some of the insane did not come from them alone. In the domestic management of the 'lunatic' we sometimes see that restraint—tying with ropes, locking in rooms—could precipitate, as much as control, violence. The *Medical Press* deplored one such case in 1873, arguing from it for the superiority of asylum care. At Ennyvale near Coleraine (Co. Derry) a 35-year-old insane woman had lived with her father, mother and sister for nearly six years. Although she was usually quiet and harmless her father always took the precaution, when leaving the house, of tying her to a stake and 'otherwise securing her' in one of the rooms. On one occasion he went out with the other daughter. They returned to find the mother murdered by the daughter who had broken loose, 'enraged at being confined', in the words of the *Medical Press*.[67] A woman admitted to the Richmond asylum in 1894 had a fractured rib and bruises. She spoke with bitterness of her brother and others at home having beaten and sat upon her. In an interview with the superintendent, her brother claimed she had been very violent and troublesome for a long time, trying to get out of windows and escape from home.

> She was particularly resistive at night & she required to be held down in bed. He said the marks on her arms and chest were caused by her being held down in bed with her hands being pressed against her chest & also that when held in this position she drummed her elbows against her chest & marked herself sometimes in that way.[68]

Judged by the complaints received at official level, women appear to have suffered more frequently than men from the practice of domestic restraint. Certainly, as we have seen, men were more likely to be committed to an asylum as 'dangerous' indicating a greater resort to the resources of the police; violence or restlessness on the part of

women, on the other hand, was evidently more readily met by a countervailing violence on the part of males in their domestic environment.[69] Examples are common.

In one case, in which the government considered prosecution, the police were asked to inquire into the alleged ill-treatment of a Leitrim woman by her husband and father-in-law. The district inspector reported that several people had testified to her having bruises about her face and body, cuts and black eyes. However, there was only one witness to an assault on her: a carman who drove the woman, her husband, brother and cousin from the station to home one night. He claimed that the brother, a Dublin constable, had struck her several times with his fists and subsequently with his umbrella which he broke on her. They had acted with 'such brutality' to her that he threatened not to drive on.[70] Since there were always difficulties about the legal status of the evidence of an asylum inmate, in this case the victim, the government decided not to prosecute. Yet the evidence of gross ill-treatment was unarguable in many cases. A 44-year-old woman with three children was admitted to the Richmond asylum with 'domestic troubles'. On examination her whole body, arms and legs were blackened and swollen with dark lines as if struck by a stick. She told the doctor that one of her sons had beaten her with a cane because she was noisy. She had to be kept in bed after admission to recover.[71] Who was persecutor and who victim was problematical indeed in many admissions preceded by violence. Mary M—, a 31-year-old mother of eight children, was admitted to the Richmond for allegedly assaulting her husband and child. She herself had a black eye caused by a blow from her husband.[72] A 60-year-old woman who had been in the asylum several times had several large bruises on her legs caused, she said, by her husband hitting her with a stick.[73] In understanding such histories we need to look beyond the asylum and its inmates to family relationships and behaviour, and perhaps not least to the impact of drink. More than one woman arriving in the asylum had reason to complain of a drinking husband.[74]

From this evidence, merely the patina of deeply troubled family relationships, we *can* see the escalation of violence and restraint leading so often to committal. But violence in itself was not the necessary precursor of asylum admission. In fact the legal process, as we have seen in Chapter 3, encouraged the presentation of evidence for it in cases where it was of minimal significance. Thus a 62-year-old Fermanagh farmer was committed to Omagh asylum after 'he made a violent assault upon his brother ... by kicking him on the leg ... while

being held by two other men'.[75] But the more substantial reason for his admission was his reported depression, sleeplessness, fears that he was losing all his means of supporting his wife and family, his 'talking foolishly' about matters with no foundation. While violence, whether to self and/or others, seemed to hold out the most obvious justification for confinement, an equally important function of the asylum was the disposal of those who had 'broken down'. The pre-histories of these breakdowns commonly involve recent or prolonged stress, commonly the loss of children, at other times failed personal relationships or 'disappointments' as the asylum terminology had it.

Substantial changes in a person's behaviour were frequently remarked as a result of personal loss. Thus Adam Carson, remanded in Belfast prison on a charge of assaulting his wife, was committed from there to the asylum in April 1891. The medical report recorded that they had lost two children from scarlet fever a few weeks before. A few days after this Carson 'began to talk strange & say he intended killing himself & family as he was tired of this world'.[76] While this man was still in the asylum twelve years later, others who were admitted subsequent to a loss frequently were discharged quickly—these cases suggest more the inadequacy (or even the absence) of relatives or friends to cope with the grief and shock of those who had lost children and spouses. A 32-year-old widow admitted to the Richmond asylum on 30 December 1891 was perhaps such a case. She had borne six children, all delivered by forceps under chloroform—five of them had died at birth. It was probably after one of these deaths that she had spent some time in the Mater Hospital the March before, 'suffering from melancholy'. Seven days before admission her husband died. On admission she had various fears about salvation and delusions about voices, but six weeks later she had 'lost' these; she was discharged at the end of March.[77] The woman arrested on the banks of the canal as a suspected suicide case was in the asylum only nine days.[78]

Some had been left isolated by loss and their resulting condition was symptomatic of this. A 50-year-old domestic servant admitted from the South Dublin Union workhouse could give a 'very good account of herself'. Although described as single on admission, she was in fact widowed. Her husband had died fifteen years before and their two children had also died very young. She dissipated her problems in drinking and after a heavy bout would go into the Union. 'She looks depressed', the doctor recorded, '& talks in a sad tone but is very coherent, intelligent & orderly.'[79] She was discharged after three and a half months. Loss of one's family was not the only source of

isolation and mourning. Another 50-year-old domestic servant, admitted for attempting to choke herself, gave an intelligent account of her history—she had been nursing her master, for whom she had worked for twenty years, and to whom she was greatly attached; after his death she 'fretted a good deal' and admitted her mind was astray. Her great fear now was that she would be kept in the asylum for the rest of her life.[80] More fortunate than most who were admitted at her age, she was discharged after eight months. Another domestic servant, admitted in October 1892, was 'very upset since her old missus died'—her well-planned retirement, for which she had saved to get her own lodgings, fell apart in suspicions of her friends 'making designs' on her.[81]

Breakdown might also come inexplicably, unattached to any obvious change in the person's environment. Thus, a schoolmaster was admitted to Sligo asylum in May 1892:

> For several months before admission he had been behaving in very strange ways, dressing in an eccentric fashion, smoking immoderately & drinking, going away to Dublin, Glasgow etc. & squandering his money—His school was going to the bad.

But in this case resort was had to an explanation in terms of family history—his father was said to have died in Swift's asylum in Dublin; a brother had been confined three or four times—and the teacher's own bad history: he had himself been in Swift's in 1879 and in 1882 had been admitted to Sligo after 'entering the bedroom of his Asst Master with a loaded revolver & threatening to shoot him'.[82] His wife this time came to see the superintendent for advice, obtained a committal form and arranged for his admission. For others the breakdown had none of these forewarnings. For instance a national school teacher who had been teaching at a small town in Mayo for nineteen years—he was married with nine children (from 11 months to 11 years); on 23 January 1906 he 'exhibited what might be termed mild symptoms of insanity'; he was kept at home in hope of recovery but only became worse and was admitted to Castlebar asylum two months later.[83] The preciseness with which the wife could recall the 'breakdown' was unusual. If the breakdown of a domestic servant—who arrived in Oslo, Norway, in February 1903 'mentally deranged'—occurred on some particular day there may well have been no one to notice it. She was an orphan who, with her sister, had been brought up by a doctor's wife in Kilrush, Co. Clare. Her sister had died after

marriage; their one brother had emigrated to America. She had been in service to the doctor and his wife for seventeen years till 1891. For seven years from then the police could discover nothing more of her history. From 1898 to May 1902 she was in service at Derry; from May to December she worked in a hotel in Carndonagh. She then returned to Derry and lived in a lodging house for three months until February 1903. During this time she was employed for only one week. She then left for Glasgow and was next heard of by the British consul in Oslo. A 'mentally deranged' woman (or man) was not a welcome addition to any country—from Norway she was sent back to Hull, whence she would be transferred to Derry or any Irish port, there to be sent to an asylum.[84] Doubtless this was, in essence, a common enough story—servants or labourers, socially isolated by the twin effects of family death and emigration, gradually worn down by the difficulty of finding or holding work, leading a marginal existence and ending in the asylum. Unfortunately in this case we have only a chronology of events and not a description of the woman herself as she moved from one workplace to another. In the following example, on the other hand, we have an unusually detailed account of a young woman's breakdown as it appeared to those around her.

Ann Garvan, an illiterate woman, sought help for her sister Eliza in 1864. She gave information before a magistrate that Eliza was a lunatic but that the family was unwilling to have her committed to prison as a dangerous lunatic—'although extremely poor [they] were quite willing to keep her' and believed she was only a danger to herself. Both women and another sister lived with their mother

> on a little Park of about a quarter of an acre of land on the mountain of Forth [near Wexford] and support ourselves by our labour ... [Eliza] was at service in Waterford and came home about two months ago and she said she was sent home—she went to Waterford a twelvemonth of last May and for a year before she went she wore a veil, which no other poor working girl about the Country did and she used to say she would be a rich lady yet.

Otherwise there was nothing 'remarkable' in her conduct before she went nor for a month after she came back. Yet she (the informant) did hear the neighbours say that ever since she returned

> she used to go into the neighbours houses talking very foolish talk and that her young Master in Waterford Mr Samuel Kent was to

marry her and got letters wrote to him and that he was to turn Catholic with her and I heard that some of the neighbours for their amusement gave her a likeness of the Prince and Princess of Wales and told her it was the likeness of her and Mr Kent.

When Eliza was told to give up the foolish thoughts of Mr Kent she took up the iron poker and threatened her sister with it. She went off to Waterford saying she was going to be married but of course returned a few days later. Her 'foolish thoughts' continued, so a friend named Paddy Tobin

> told her in my presence that young Mr Kent was dead and that a memory was to be held over him and he pretended to read it for her from the newspaper for the purpose of trying to put the notion ... out of her head, but instead of that she became quite frantic and ran out on the door and I heard her say she would put an end to herself.[85]

The amateur attempt by Paddy Tobin to remove her 'foolish thoughts' by removing the source of them has some interesting parallels in one conception of the role of the asylum: to remove the inmate from disturbing features of his or her social environment. Eliza Garvan was not considered out of her mind in wearing a veil, though nobody else did—but when she persisted with her fantasies of marrying her master she was clearly 'foolish'. But perhaps they were not fantasies. Possibly she had been deceived by the master. A notorious example from 1869 illustrates the possibility.

On 19 June in that year Marian Slater, a 24-year-old Protestant (the religion here is relevant) servant was committed to Carlow asylum for hysteria—a condition 'to which almost any female is liable', thought an inspector of lunatics. From the time of her committal the resident and visiting physicians and the Protestant chaplain considered her collected and rational, free of delusions. In fact, thought the superintendent, Dr Howlett, she should not have been admitted to the asylum at all. In subsequent investigations it emerged that she had been engaged to a policeman she met while working in Athy; when she had to move to a new situation in Co. Cork she had corresponded with him and sent him money. While she was away he 'transferred his affections to another'; later he wrote a letter saying he was in hospital seriously ill (the motivation for this letter was not clear; perhaps to get more money, or a prelude to breaking their engagement). She left her employment in Cork as a result of

receiving this letter and returned to Athy. There she found that he had deceived her—he was not ill at all, he was with another woman, and was a Catholic, not a Protestant as he had told her. In a confrontation with the policeman and the new woman she became very excited and said that he made her mad enough to commit suicide. At this he took her to the police station where the head constable kept her in custody for the night (the latter explained later that he considered her 'too respectable to send to jail'). Released the next morning, she stayed with the family of a friend. When she continued to be excited and threatened suicide the friend (also a servant) swore an information to have her committed. She was discharged from the asylum within a month, following a report on the case by Inspector Nugent. Subsequently the constable was dismissed from the service for deceiving his superiors in the course of their investigation of the incident.[86] The ill-treatment this woman received, the 'manufacture' of her madness, the manipulation of the law by a policeman who was personally interested—all this was not typical. Rather it was one of those confinements of convenience which always worried the defenders of personal liberty in campaigns against madhouses. The certification of this domestic servant was certainly unwarranted in contemporary eyes. Yet there is but a fine distinction between her actions—excited, hysterical, verbally threatening suicide, perhaps threatening the policeman and his new associate (her friend thought she might do 'bodily harm' to them)—between this catalogue of behaviours and similar ones in so many other committals to the asylum.

Mania and melancholia, the two great categories of nineteenth-century psychiatric classification, were made to encompass a wide range of symptoms and behaviours. As the wiser asylum doctors recognised, they were relatively useless labels disguising the varied histories and prognoses of those committed to the asylum.

The Family

Underlying the cases we have cited have been not just varying manifestations of behaviour, violent and otherwise; or incapacity to support oneself (equally the inadequacy of social supports) in old age, idiocy or through the process of temporary or permanent breakdown—we have also touched tangentially on the family context of most of these examples. The family might be merely the setting for an unaccountable change in a person's life, a change which other

members of the family could only describe as going 'out of his/her mind'. But we have also seen instances in which the insanity of the person committed was symptomatic of the conflict within the family. The elements of this conflict were varied. To some extent, given the inadequacies of the evidence, they are undiscoverable. Yet what does stand out in this evidence is the centrality of the family as the context of madness, where the 'derangement' is expressed and where it is defined as such. We need to remember the exceptions to this—the workhouse in particular, a prolific source of asylum inmates, and a place where one sees the most blatant examples of institutional expediency in certifying troublesome people. There is also the case of those whose aggression was directed indiscriminately against the outside world—Peter Smith, who hit a farmer who did not know him, splitting his forehead with a shovel; Alexander McArthur, who assaulted several children in a public school in Co. Antrim and who five years previously had assaulted a man in Kilrea (Derry) while 'wandering about a stranger'; or Patrick Hanrahan, a Limerick labourer, who was certified after smashing 'fifty-two panes of Glass in the window of the Parish Church at Kilfinane' in 1857.[87] There were a certain number of such cases every year. But the greater number of committals originated in the family home—one relative, a parent, child, sister or brother, perhaps an uncle or aunt, swore an information before the justice and sought the help of the police in taking one of the family to the asylum. In concluding this account of the social context of insane behaviour we will explore the dimensions of the family's place in the process of 'going mad'. What we are interested in is the way in which, in Roger Bastide's terms, predisposition (from whatever cause) is acted out in a social context which furthers the tendency of the predisposition.[88]

The possibility of going out of one's mind existed almost as a threat in some families;[89] equally there was the threat of making a member of the family mad, that is by sending him or her to the asylum. A young woman, discharged a few days before, was brought back to the Richmond asylum in August 1892—'she states herself that her mother sent her back here as she refused to work at home, she did not do work as she was "not inclined" '.[90] A house painter, admitted on a charge of threatening to kill his wife and to cut his own throat, did not appear at any time during his two months stay in the asylum 'to be insane'. His story remained consistent throughout this time—in consequence of the dirty and neglected way his wife kept his children, he often went out at night; whenever he remonstrated with his wife she

'threatened' to put him in the asylum; on 27 September he sought to 'reason cases' with her; he got excited and may have used wild threats without meaning to do harm. His wife then had him committed.[91] In this way the threat of violence could be met by the threat of certification.

The use of the asylum, or the threat of it, as an instrument of control in the family could be quite blatant. A young slater's assistant, apparently living with his parents, was committed for threatening to cut his father's throat, having a razor, and 'delusions'. On admission he smelled of whiskey, seemed to be recovering from a drunken bout, but was quite rational and coherent. A few days before, he said, he tried to separate his father and mother in a family quarrel; both were drunk. They subsequently swore informations against him and, in his words, 'had him sent here to teach him a lesson'. A week after admission his father came to take him out on bail; questioned by the doctor, he corroborated the son's story. He

> moreover assured me that at no time did he consider his son insane, but that he thought it would do him [the son] good to get a few days here.[92]

In the statements of the insane we frequently see *their* consciousness of this sort of thing—unfortunately we do not usually have the evidence (as in the above case) from the other side. Thus a young woman was admitted to the Richmond in 1892: six years ago, she says, she was sent to a private asylum for refusing to go to school.[93] Sophia T—, a 42-year-old single woman who died just over a month after admission, said she was sent in because 'her people were anxious to get shut of her', a phrase which vividly evokes her exclusion.[94] She also had been in an asylum before. To send a discharged lunatic back to the asylum was inevitably a threat which could be used to control her when at home.

Other events demonstrated the use of madness as a means by which one member of a family could account for and then attempt to control the unacceptable behaviour of another. Let us consider three such cases. In 1859 the owner of a whiskey shop complained in a memorial to the Lord-Lieutenant that the proprietor of a private lunatic asylum in Limerick allowed his wife to escape in order to reap the benefit from the remaining quarter's maintenance which was already paid. He wanted her to be re-committed. When she was admitted, the proprietor reported, Mrs Cooney was perfectly rational, though

having been certified by two medical men; she was suffering from the effects of delirium tremens and he had to wean her off porter while she was there; she had several 'contusions' on her body and a severe mark on her wrist which she said was caused by her husband—'when he got drunk she mentioned he was most violent'. The female attendant who went to the house the day after the escape found Mrs Cooney going 'about her household duties quietly and rationally'. And her daughter expressed her own embarrassment at the course of events since there was an element of public shame attached to the committal of a relative to an asylum. She did not want her mother to be taken back to the asylum as 'it would make a show of the family to press on her to go back'. On the other hand, the husband's brother who had assisted in putting her in the asylum claimed that she was 'ten times worse in every respect than before [her committal]'. Perhaps she was; but this, given her mild state with the attendant and her daughter, only indicated her antagonism to those who had confined her.[95] The evidence suggested the alcoholism of both husband and wife; but within this family it was the former, with his brother, who defined the madness of the latter.

Similarly a clerk in the Grand Canal Company wanted his wife placed under 'proper control' by the authorities until her 'mental condition' improved. His request unveils very neatly a set of popular presumptions about behaviour and normality and their relation to 'mental condition'. As he tells the story she had left home some months before after 14 years' marriage, 'her mind having become unsound'; she went from Dublin to stay in Belfast where he got two medical men to see her (one of them was her brother); they declared she was mentally deranged, but they would not put her under restraint as 'they thought moral suasion might help to restore her balance'. She came back to Dublin but refused to live with her husband, and stayed in an apartment for two weeks, then went to Arklow where she had been for a couple of months. We are then told that when she sees *him* she becomes worse. Her insanity he says is due to her indulgence in drink. A police report from Arklow later throws another light on her behaviour. While agreeing that drink is probably the cause of 'the peculiarity in her manner' the head constable concludes that she is apparently well able to take care of herself.

> Beyond a certain reserve in her manner, a silence in disposition and a disinclination to be interviewed by the police there was no indication of mental derangement in her demeanour.

Thus at each remove from this woman a different perception of her behaviour was held—to her husband she was insane and became worse when she saw him; to the doctors she was mentally deranged but not certifiable, indeed even amenable to 'moral suasion'; to the police, she merely had a peculiarity in her manner.[96]

The husband's role was again the focus of attention in a court case in 1897 in which a woman sued her stepfather for maintenance for her mother—she had supported the latter for three years previously. Her case rested on his ill-treatment of her mother. Moreover, she claimed that he had committed her to Armagh asylum in 1893, when she was 'perfectly in her senses'. She had taken the mother out of the asylum after six weeks and thereafter supported her in Belfast. While the asylum doctors considered her admission justified—'she used very filthy and abominable language and conducted herself in an insane manner'; she had been drinking heavily and this, they considered, may have produced her behaviour—the judge described the committal as a farce. Only one doctor had certified her (two were required for 'private' patients) and, the judge held, there was no evidence of mental disorder on the certificate which stated:

> Violent & using most threatening language and swearing at her husband and having broken several panes of glass in various rooms.[97]

It avoided mentioning her two black eyes (noted by the asylum staff on her admission), thus disguising the husband's role in the domestic conflict.

As these three cases suggest, madness existed to the extent that some person other than the lunatic defined it as such. Thus it could be the expression of violent or conflict-ridden social relations in which the dominance of one over the other was the origin of committal. The reasons brought to justify the committal suggested the cultural values and expectations which defined normal behaviour. A 25-year-old woman who was violent to her parents was committed to the Omagh asylum in 1871; her condition was described as having an 'aversion to her mother'. The 'form of mental disorder' in a 19-year-old male inmate was a 'desire to leave home'. The only grounds given by the father of a 17-year-old labourer were that 'he has repeatedly wandered away from home and was away from the 18 July 1891 till the 29th July 1891'.[98] Charlotte, a 26-year-old single woman, re-admitted to the Richmond asylum for violently assaulting her mother, expressed her frustration at her mother's dominance:

the only thing she has against her mother is that after buying her new things, the mother brays and boasts of it, saying that she is too indulgent to [her].[99]

In this way everyday conflicts of 'children' (in their late adolescence and twenties) were translated into forms of madness.

The history of family conflict was revealed further in instances where one relative intervened to defend the insane member from another. This was usually a brother or a sister. We have considered some of these interventions earlier—a brother contesting the insanity of his sister whom he argued should not be in an asylum as she was only suffering from a puerperal fever; or the brother of George McClean, who tried to take him out of the Omagh asylum, against the wishes of McClean's wife.[100] In the latter case, after McClean was discharged, he went to live with his brother. In 1897, Arthur Warner of Scilly (near Kinsale, Co. Cork) was found unfit to plead to a charge of assault against his wife and was sent to Cork asylum. Subsequently there were two appeals by his sister, who lived about a mile away from their home at Scilly, for his discharge. The superintendent considered he would be dangerous to his wife if he lived with her again, but thought he might be able to live with his sister. In a curious sequel to this recommendation, the police inspector at Bandon (where the wife was staying) reported that Mrs Warner did not oppose his discharge as long as she had security that he would not interfere with her; she refused to live with him. But the police inspector at Kinsale thought that the superintendent's suggestion would be dangerous.

Warner's sister lives about a mile from where Mrs Warner lives & is suspected of being in a good measure the cause of the quarrels between Warner & his wife.

She apparently wanted to get her sister-in-law out of the house; because 'it belongs to her brother [she says] that Mrs Warner has no claim for it'.

If Warner is released I believe the family disputes will be as bad as ever & no one can know with what result.

The news of Warner's impending release had meanwhile been 'leaked' and the residents of this little community prepared a petition against his discharge. He was, in their opinion, a 'dangerous

homicidal maniac'; his sister was an old and feeble woman who would be unable to control him. Warner was not released.[101]

Particularly in small rural communities the state of family relations could be well known and, as the above case illustrates, the concern of neighbours as well as relatives. In a similar way, an 'escaped lunatic' became the object of community contentions in 1905. This man's wife wrote to the Ballinasloe superintendent asking for him to be retaken:

> he is still hovering from here to Drum and Moore [*sic*] I see no sign of getting him back. It is now time to prepare to sow something to eat for the Children no man no matter who he is will work one day on the land while he is hovering about they dread him.

She claimed that the police were taking his side, as he had been seen a couple of times in the area but not recaptured. Whether or not the police were tardy in pursuing him was difficult to say, but a police report indicates that he had many friends who were ready to help him. As well, the asylum superintendent reported that people in the area gave contradicitory opinions about the cause of his committal; some supported his wife, others the man's denial that he had threatened her and the children. His state of temper with her was not improved when she attempted to have their farm transferred to her name.[102]

One last example of this extension of family conflicts: a Belfast tradesman was admitted with 'acute melancholia' after a suicide attempt. He was discharged to the care of his father on his brother's application but re-admitted a few months later after moving back with his wife. Within some weeks she was writing to the Belfast asylum opposing her brother-in-law's attempts to have him discharged again:

> I am in downright terror of him so I hope you will not allow him to be taken out again he may work a little while but then he stops and then he comes to bother me. He attempted his own life twice before, and his brother and father are nearly as bad as himself. I am in a good situation and well thought of but no one would have him coming about, I had to leave my last place on account of him.

The brother persisted (from Glasgow) with his efforts to have his discharged. He claimed that the wife had got 'up a false charge'; that he was a good tradesman and had got a good position in Glasgow last time he was discharged.

I think it is a great shame that a man of his ability should be confined in an asylum because his wife refuses to live with him.

(Or, he could have added, because *her* employers would not put up with him.) Although the inmate had not 'recovered' the superintendent agreed that he could be discharged to his brother.[103] In such a way could detention or discharge be determined. Life outside the asylum was possible for an 'unrecovered' lunatic; but it did depend on the social context in which that life would be carried on.

The details of these few histories show us some of the complexities behind those brief statements we find in case-books and inspectors' reports—a soldier admitted to the Richmond who described the case of his depression, 'various family troubles'; a young domestic servant whose 'anxiety' centred on her failure to get on with her sisters; Foley, a Kerry tailor, previously in the Killarney asylum, who hanged himself from a rafter in his kitchen after his wife had gone to Killorglin petty sessions to prosecute him for assault—from April to October 1875 he was fit for discharge but his wife refused to have him back. The asylum superintendent had no doubt he was sane on leaving the asylum but considered that ... 'unhappy differences with his family which appear to have been of long duration quickly brought on a relapse'.[104] It is evident that the insane, that is those committed to the asylum, could as equally be victims as dangers within family structures. Some threatened violence, some even used it. But it was also the case that the insane were the objects of violence, particularly if they were women. And the lunacy committal was in many hands an instrument of domination, to reinforce a position of power in the family or an expectation of certain behaviour. Where its use was not so blatant as this, it was bound up with a set of cultural expectations that the asylum was now, by the end of the nineteenth century, the appropriate place for those who were 'out of their mind'; they might even recover there. This value could be internalised even by one who was 'out of his senses'. We are told by the informant that John Little, a Tyrone labourer, 'threatened ... that he would do injury if he was not taken to the Asylum where he said that he would get better'.[105]

From the statistics of asylum admissions we can draw the most general conclusions about the common social characteristics of the insane—the tendency to such high admissions among those in their thirties, the slightly higher number of males committed, the much greater propensity of the single to be admitted and so on. But it is evident from the substance of this chapter that there was an immense

variety of behaviour and contexts within which madness was perceived. When some early-nineteenth-century asylum reformers (indeed founders) talked of the lunatics they were going to house, they were, for the most part, ignorant of the material they were acting on. The historiography of the asylum has usually followed them—there has been little attempt to explore the social meanings and determinants of madness in the nineteenth century.[106] The epithet, 'the insane', does not sufficiently characterise the quality of the interaction of these people with a 'sane society' in which they had frequently lived and worked in ways no different from those who never saw the inside of an asylum. From their histories, it emerges that some survived their exclusion from the sane world to return to an uncertain, though not always bleak, future. Others were the worst casualties of hard times, subject to repeated blows of economic, social and personal misfortune: many of these finished their lives in the asylum. In the following chapter we will examine the experience of both these groups in the asylum.

Notes

1. Sean O'Casey, *Drums under the Windows* (Autobiography, Book 3) (Pan, London, 1972) pp. 47-65 (first published 1945). The incident is dated pre-1914.

2. J.M. Synge, *Collected Works Volume II Prose* (Oxford University Press, London, 1966), pp. 209-11, 216-20 (in the collection of pieces entitled, 'In Wicklow, West Kerry and Connemara').

3. 'Census of Paupers, 31st March 1906', pp. 19-21, in *Royal Commission on the Poor Laws*, Appendix to the tenth volume of evidence, *HC* (1910), l.

4. All references to statistical details of the asylum population are taken from the annual reports of the inspectors of lunatics.

5. The general facts of delayed or avoided marriage in the post-Famine period are beyond dispute though the interpretation of them has been a matter of some debate. See, in particular, the papers by the late K.H. Connell, 'Peasant Marriage in Ireland: its Structure and Development since the Famine', *Economic History Review (EHR)*, 2nd ser., vol. 14 (1961), pp. 502-23, and 'Catholicism and Marriage in the Century after the Famine' in his *Irish Peasant Society* (Clarendon Press, Oxford, 1968); Brendan M. Walsh, 'Marriage Rates and Population Pressure: Ireland, 1871 and 1911', *EHR*, 2nd ser., vol. 23 (1970), pp. 148-62; and Robert E. Kennedy, Jr., *The Irish: Emigration, Marriage, and Fertility* (University of California Press, Berkeley, California, 1973).

6. Two recent anthropological accounts have emphasised the relation between demographic decline, social isolation and problems of mental illness and alcoholism in contemporary rural Ireland. See Hugh Brody, *Inishkillane: Change and Decline in the West of Ireland* (Penguin, Harmondsworth, 1973), pp. 86-108 and Nancy Scheper-Hughes, *Saints, Scholars and Schizophrenics: Mental Illness in Rural Ireland* (University of California Press, Berkeley, 1979), pp. 34-40, 53-8.

7. In the category 'immediate relative' I have included wife, husband, father, mother or sibling. A number of other admissions in each year had an aunt, uncle or cousin at the

same address. The proportions for 'immediate relative' for each year (with surviving warrants out of total admissions in brackets) are:

1861	1871	1881	1891	1901
83%	81%	82%	83%	74%
(86/?146)	(133/160)	(128/129)	(153/156)	(175/177)

Source: HOS 29/1/5/601-7200, PRONI.

8. *Transactions of the National Association for the Promotion of Social Science* (1858), p. 517.

9. RP 1891/23052.

10. Richmond District Lunatic Asylum, Male Case-Book, 1852-80, p. 9 (hereafter these case-books are referred to as RMCB, males; RFCB, females).

11. *Report*, p. 47, *HC* (1846), xxii; *14th Report* p. 27, *HC* (1865), xxi.

12. *10th Report*, p. 6, *HC* (1861), xxvii; *15th Report*, p. 9, *HC* (1866), xxxii; *Report*, p. 47, *HC* (1846), xxii. For the criticism of the asylums' spartan conditions see *Royal Commission*, p. 22, *HC* (1857-8), xxvii. For the asylum as an agent of social improvement of the 'humbler classes' see below, p. 183.

13. See Dermot Walsh and Brendan Walsh, 'Mental Illness in the Republic of Ireland—First Admissions', *Journal of the Irish Medical Association*, vol. 63, no. 400 (1970), pp. 365-70. This study strongly supported the hypothesis that regional variation in hospitalisation rates in Ireland was a function of the country's abnormal demographic structure. It did not present data for any period earlier than the 1960s but the judgement about the nineteenth-century situation presumably draws on the statistics in Dermot Walsh, 'Hospitalized Psychiatric Morbidity in the Republic of Ireland', *British Journal of Psychiatry*, vol. 114 (1968), pp. 11-14.

14. *Report*, p. 37, *HC* (1847), xvii.

15. *MPC*, Irish Supplement, 26 August 1914.

16. Cf. F.G. Crookshank, 'The Frequency of Phthithis Pulmonalis in Asylums ...', *JMS*, vol. 45 (1899), pp. 657-83.

17. *JMS*, vol. 39 (1893), pp. 308-11, for Conolly Norman's comment on a paper on general paralysis of the insane. His impression is confirmed by mortality statistics. In 1905 the relative proportions (per cent) of all public asylum deaths caused by general paralysis in Britain and Ireland were:

	England and Wales	Scotland	Ireland
Males	26·4	22·5	5·3
Females	7·4	7·0	1·1

Source: the annual reports of the lunacy authorities in each country for 1905, *HC* (1906), xxxviii and xxxix.

18. *MPC*, Irish Supplement, 7 December 1892.

19. *MPC*, Irish Supplement, 22 February 1882.

20. RP 1891/23052.

21. RP 1895/8093.

22. *Freeman's Journal*, 6 January 1862; for a similar case see *Irish Times*, 23 May 1862 (both in Larcom Papers, NLI, MS. 7776).

23. *MPC*, 14 November 1900.

24. RP 1864/21068.

25. RP 1872/12214.

26. *20th Report*, p. 7, *HC* (1871), xxvi.

27. RFCB (1891-2), pp. 409, 509, 437, 533. Tuberculosis, commonly associated with asylum committals (in part perhaps due to the restlessness and anxiety produced in its later stages) was another factor which probably made women more vulnerable to this use of the asylum. It was a greater cause of mortality among females in Irish asylums than among males (by about 5 per cent in 1901 and 1911). It has been argued that the high incidence of tuberculosis mortality among women in nineteenth-century Britain and Ireland reflected their disadvantaged social position, specifically through their poorer nutrition relative to male members of households: cf. Sheila Ryan

Johansson, 'Sex and Death in Victorian England' in Martha Vicinus (ed.), *A Widening Sphere: Changing Roles of Victorian Women* (Indiana University Press, Bloomington, 1977), pp. 163-81, and Robert E. Kennedy, Jr., *The Irish: Emigration, Marriage and Fertility* (University of California Press, Berkeley, California, 1973), pp. 41-65.

28. *MPC*, Irish Supplement, 1 November 1911 and 3 January 1912; ibid., 21 September 1904 reporting the 74th Annual Report of the Belfast District Lunatic Asylum.

29. *MPC*, Irish Supplement, 18 December 1903.

30. RP 1893/11888.

31. RP 1883/21861. Keith Thomas has pointed to the particular vulnerability to charges of witchcraft of the socially dependent, particularly old women, in sixteenth- and seventeenth-century English villages. There too the phenomenon must be seen against the 'breakdown of the tradition of mutual help upon which many English village communities were based'. Keith Thomas, 'The Relevance of Social Anthropology to the Historical Study of English Witchcraft' in Mary Douglas (ed.), *Witchcraft Confessions and Accusations*, (Tavistock, London, 1970), pp. 63-4, and *Religion and the Decline of Magic*, (Penguin, Harmondsworth, 1973), pp. 673-7.

32. RP 1876/19445, and 1876/15913. *MPC*, Irish Supplement, 1 November 1911.

33. RP 1888/5486.

34. RP 1872/11461.

35. RP 1898/6177.

36. *19th Report*, p. 27, *HC* (1870), xxxiv.

37. Ibid., p. 38.

38. See the evidence relating to the Stewart institution in *Royal Commission on the Care and Control of the Feeble-Minded*, Minutes of Evidence, vol. III, *HC* (1908), xxxviii. Sir Christopher Nixon (ev. 22555) noted that the Archbishop of Dublin, Dr Walsh, had offered to set up a Catholic home on the lines of the Stewart institution but this had not eventuated by the time of the commission's hearings.

39. RP 1877/827.

40. *MPC*, Irish Supplement, 17 August 1904.

41. For the difficulties in the way of establishing compulsory treatment of chronic alcoholics see Roy M. MacLeod, 'The Edge of Hope: Social Policy and Chronic Alcoholism 1870-1900', *Journal of the History of Medicine and Allied Sciences*, vol. 22 (1967), pp. 215-45. As in England, there was little response in Ireland to the Inebriates Act of 1898 (61 & 62 Vic., c. 60). Not before 1905 was an inspector of retreats and certified inebriate reformatories appointed for Ireland (G.P. O'Farrell, the inspector of lunatics). The only facilities provided under the Act were 'The Lodge Inebriate Retreat, Belfast' founded by the Irish Women's Temperance Union in 1902 and brought under the Act in 1903 so that inmates could be detained; a state inebriate reformatory at Ennis which was actually under the general prisons board; and certified inebriate reformatories at Waterford (1906) and Wexford (1909), founded by Catholic religious orders. By the time of the last report of the Irish inspector (*HC*, 1920, xviii) both the Waterford and Wexford reformatories had closed. RP 1907/10901, RP 1901/7589, RP 1910/15946 and RP 1918/5058. Teetotalers may have, as Brian Harrison suggests in *Drink and the Victorians* (Faber, London, 1971), p. 365 'helped to substitute compassion for condemnation' in social attitudes to the drunkard but such a change failed to make itself felt in the area of treatment of alcoholism. Doubtless the problems were partly financial, partly the failure of the advocates of treatment to prove that successful treatment was possible. Moreover, there was the problem of detaining people who had not committed a crime and, when sober at least, were as 'sane' as anybody else. And there was also the widespread survival of an attitude which found the drunkard largely responsible for his own condition and therefore liable to punishment rather than treatment.

42. RP 1901/7825.

43. RP 1897/19870.

44. RP 1872/15831.

45. RP 1897/3629.

46. RP 1873/11736.

47. RMCB (1852-80), p. 85.

48. *MPC*, Irish Supplement, 12 February 1896.

49. Thus the Limerick governors—'the affliction to which it has pleased Providence to afflict [the insane]'; RP 1845/G8338, encl. 1844/G3732. 'Through God's inscrutable providence', a petitioner writes to the Lord-Lieutenant, his friend has been 'deprived of reason'; RP 1848/G5433. Not long since, according to the *Dublin Evening Post* in 1856, 'Insanity was regarded as a terrible and mysterious visitation of Providence for which there was no cure—no relief', *MPC*, 8 October 1856. A mother writes of her daughter that 'it pleased God to Afflict [her] with Insanity'; RP 1877/9423. The agents of medical treatment themselves did not surrender this explanation by act of Providence. Dr Woods of Cork wishes in 1881 to 'separate visitations of Providence [i.e. insanity] from vicious acts [i.e. crime]'; *MPC*, 6 April 1881. An inspector of lunatics describes a patient's restlessness in 1901 as 'the direct result of the particular form of mental disturbance with which it has pleased Providence to afflict him'; RP 1901/9759.

50. D. Walsh, 'A Century of Suicide in Ireland', *Journal of the Irish Medical Association*, vol. 69 (1976), pp. 144-52.

51. RMCB (1888-9), p. 145.

52. Ibid., p. 161.

53. RMCB (1852-80), p. 381.

54. RFCB (1889-91), p. 517.

55. Ibid., p. 597. Cf. ibid., p. 329 for a woman who went down to the Liffey one night 'after taking too much drink, was going to thrown herself in, on the prompting of the Devil, when some people passing by asked what she was doing and told her to go home'.

56. Ibid., p. 341.

57. RP 1901/3092.

58. RP 1876/3167. The relative of another Omagh inmate makes the same complaint. The writer says that the doctors hold out no hope for improvement and therefore she wants the woman released—'Had I known when she was admitted, that there would be any difficulty in obtaining her discharge if she showed no signs of improvement, I should never have given her up.' HOS 29/1/5/3665.

59. RP 1911/10264.

60. RP 1882/45212.

61. RP 1862/18258.

62. RP 1908/19623.

63. Cf. RP 1899/8170—a widow deprived of her only support, a son who is in Castlebar asylum; RP 1873/4139—a mother for her son, her principal support; RMCB (1905-6), p. 49—a wife for her husband, because she and her children are dependent on him.

64. RP 1846/G8680.

65. *MPC*, 20 July 1887; RP 1873/4734.

66. RP 1859/2468.

67. *MPC*, 23 April 1873.

68. RP 1894/15224.

69. See above, p. 101.

70. RP 1905/22448.

71. RFCB (1891-2), p. 205.

72. Ibid., p. 277.

73. Ibid., p. 581.

74. For such a case, see ibid., p. 277.

75. HOS 29/1/5/5221.

76. RP 1903/10397.

77. RFCB (1891-2), p. 185.

78. See above, p. 152.

79. RFCB (1891-2), p. 357. The awareness of isolation and loss is graphically amalgamated with acute despair at her own worth in another Richmond case: a single woman, 'frightfully depressed', almost blind and describing herself as 'hunch-back'— her mother died in the Mullingar asylum, her father 'of decline', as also a sister; another sister went to America; she herself appeared to have kept house for her third sister and her husband. One day in the last few months of her life somebody records her words— 'My poor body and soul is dead, tis indeed, tis indeed, tis indeed, Jane is in heaven, my mother, father—Pat and all are in Heaven, they had masses for their souls, but my soul is in Hell. I must be buried body & bones alive I must be put in a hole & buried at the back of a ditch ... Oh wouldn't I give thousands and thousands of pounds to get forgiveness but no, I am a devil, a devil, a devil & there is no hope—no hope.' Ibid., p. 753.

80. Ibid., p. 449.

81. Ibid., p. 853.

82. RP 1892/16168.

83. RP 1908/16045.

84. RP 1903/7111.

85. RP 1864/14770.

86. RP 1869/15878; *19th Report*, p. 12, *HC* (1870), xxxiv.

87. RP 1865/3022, 1877/2936, 1857/5578.

88. R. Bastide, *The Sociology of Mental Disorder* (Routledge and Kegan Paul, London, 1972), pp. 176-84. There has been more work on the changing demographic features of family structures and marriage patterns in post-Famine Ireland than on the consequences of these for social behaviour and relationships. Nevertheless, some of the stresses and conflicts arising within the family context during this period of great change are suggested by the studies of Arensberg and Kimball, Connell and Kennedy among others: the constant loss by emigration of those children not favoured with the inheritance or dowry; the tension between those who remained, particularly between the inheriting son and ageing parents who still controlled the farm, or between the old and the young after the transfer of the land; the male dominance of rural society in which women were disadvantaged even at the cost of their life expectancy; the sense of loss and isolation following from the massive rural population decline. Within Ireland, an urban centre like Dublin may have offered escape from some of these situations (particularly for young, single women, Kennedy argues) but it, in turn, presented all the stresses posed by an over-crowded, poor and economically stagnant city. See Conrad M. Arensberg and Solon T. Kimball, *Family and Community in Ireland* (2nd edn) (Harvard University Press, Cambridge, Mass., 1968), esp. chs. 6 and 7; K.H. Connell, 'Peasant Marriage in Ireland: its Structure and Development since the Famine', esp. pp. 514-18; Robert Kennedy, Jr., *The Irish*, esp. chs. III and IV; and the references in note 6 above. Cf. also Dermot Walsh, 'Two and Two Make Five—Multi-factoriogenesis in Mental Illness in Ireland', *Journal of the Irish Medical Association*, vol. 69, no. 16 (1976), pp. 417-22, on the necessity for family studies in exploring the determination of the contemporary incidence of mental illness in Ireland.

89. See above, pp. 153-4.

90. RFCB (1891-2), p. 741.

91. RMCB (1888-9), p. 297.

92. Ibid., p. 309.

93. RFCB (1891-2), p. 789.

94. Ibid., p. 845.

95. RP 1859/610.

96. RP 1907/6563.

97. RP 1897/3824; *Freeman's Journal*, 27 January 1897.

98. HOS 29/1/5/3619, 1044, 5231.

99. RFCB (1891-2), p. 125.

100. See above p. 155.

101. RP 1900/7786.

102. RP 1905/5935.

103. RP 1908/3528.

104. RMCB (1888-9), p. 377; RFCB (1891-2), p. 721; RP 1875/19963.

105. HOS 29/1/5/3675; cf. RMCB (1905-6), p. 2 for a man who 'entreated to be at once admitted to the asylum as he would commit suicide if he were not'.

106. The most recent work, published since this chapter was written, has started to amend this. Scull, *Museums of Madness: The Social Organization of Insanity in Nineteenth-Century England* (Allen Lane, London, 1979), explores the ideology of the asylum and the changing perceptions of its function in nineteenth-century England, though on a level which tends to ignore the patients. Richard W. Fox, *So far disordered in mind: Insanity in California 1870-1930* (University of California Press, Berkeley, 1978), has systematically examined a long run of commitment records to locate the social context of lunacy committals: even in the more mobile, migrant society of California the family was central to the committal process, see ibid., pp. 96-8. See also John K. Walton, 'Lunacy in the Industrial Revolution: A Study of Asylum Admissions in Lancashire, 1848-50', *Journal of Social History*, vol. 13, no. 1 (1979), pp. 1-22.

5 THE ASYLUM: CUSTODY, TREATMENT, CONTROL

'The uniform tendency of all asylums', the inspectors of lunatics warned as early as 1851, 'is to degenerate from their original object, that of being hospitals for the treatment of insanity, into domiciles for incurable lunatics'.[1] When a Dublin coachman was admitted to the asylum after an attempted suicide in 1888 the doctor recorded that he 'fancies people are telling him that he is going to be put into a dead house and buried alive'.[2] His fancies rudely described a reality of confinement in the later years of the century. By 1901 nearly as many people were dying each year in the asylums of Ireland as were discharged from them. Over half of the 1,257 who died in the asylums in 1901 had been inmates for longer than two years, one in three for more than five years.[3] For many, an asylum was not just the place where they went to die but probably the immediate cause of their death. The lunatic asylums had become agents of disease. 'Asylum dysentery', various fevers and tuberculosis of the lungs were common causes of death. The Richmond asylum, for instance, had four outbreaks of beri-beri between 1894 and 1898.[4] The extravagant optimism of the 1840s and 1850s vanished in the face of the onslaught of 'incurables' who filled the asylums and made nonsense of the title, 'hospital for the insane', which some of them had adopted. In this respect, however, the asylum merely shared in the general failure of hospitals throughout much of the nineteenth century. And death at the end of a long or short stay in the asylum was not the only experience of those who were committed.

The other experience—that of a minority of admissions, but a significant one—was discharge from the asylum following a stay of some months. Thus, during 1901 when over 3,700 people were admitted to public asylums in Ireland, 1,303 were discharged. Over half of those discharged had been confined less than six months; over 80 per cent less than one year.[5] However, the history of those who were discharged was an ambiguous one. Re-admission ('relapse' in the official statistics) was common and hundreds of admissions each year were of those who had been in two, three or more times before. The criteria for discharge were not identical with those for 'recovery'. Institutional convenience or the wishes of relatives also played their part.[6] Nevertheless, there were two distinct patterns of experience

here; in deterministic fashion the medical men saw them as the experience of the 'curable' and the 'incurable'. The 'curable' were those who demonstrated good potential for early discharge. The 'incurable', on the other hand, were condemned by their constitution or by the 'advanced' state of their disease to a long, usually permanent, residence in the asylum. Such an interpretation was in itself an admission from the start of the asylum's limitations. It was an acceptance and a warning of the institution's custodial function for the majority of its inmates. But it also reflected a particular relationship between the doctors and their patients, one in which it was the former who were the ultimate arbiters of the latter's fitness to re-enter society 'at large'.

It is that nexus which we wish to explore. Within the asylum what sort of relationships existed between doctors, staff (first known as 'attendants', later as 'mental nurses') and the lunatic inmates? What was the aim of asylum treatment and by what means was it put into effect? What effect did institutional life have on the inmates and what can be said of their responses to the asylum? We will examine these questions, looking first at the structure of authority in the asylum and its ideological foundation, and secondly at the inmates' experiences of the asylum, of treatment, management and punishment.

The Asylum Hierarchy

Although the public asylums of Ireland were originally managed by laymen, 'moral governors', we have seen that the medical men took over from the 1840s. Appealing to the authority of 'medical science', but relying also on their superior capacity for organisation and political influence, the asylum doctors gradually established their control over the physical and moral treatment of their patients, a control which extended over all aspects of asylum life. In theory at least, the medical superintendent was possessed of autocratic authority over his staff, keepers, attendants, nurses, and the whole range of institutional employees, cooks, cleaners, carpenters, plumbers and so on, who made up the world of the asylum. 'The whole house', John Conolly had argued in 1847, 'every great and every trifling argument, the disposition of every officer and servant should be in perpetual conformity to his [the superintendent's] views; so that one uniform idea may animate all to whom his orders are entrusted, and the result be one uniform plan ... The manners and language of all who are

employed in the asylum should but reflect his.'[7] This totalitarian ideal was impossible to achieve; but where they could the asylum doctors sought to eliminate potential opposition to their authority within the institutions.

Although, for example, the visiting physicians retained their office until the 1890s in Ireland (nearly half a century longer than in England), their influence after the 1860s was minimal.[8] Just as the 'alienists' had subordinated the lay managers and the non-resident physicians, they also made sure in the 1850s and 1860s that the matrons in charge of the female wards would no longer be autonomous. This campaign involved an attack on the *sex* of matrons as well as on their relative independence from resident physicians. Thus an anonymous correspondent to the *Dublin Journal of Medical Science* (which promoted the asylum doctors' cause) wrote in 1857 of the evils of having 'lady-matrons' exercising powers in their divisions independent of the authority of the physician. A few pages later, commenting on the state of the Irish private asylums, he was 'happy to add [that] none are conducted by *females*, as in the case of similar establishments in England and Scotland'. Commenting on the 1858 royal commission's report the same journal suggested that the office of matron should cease and be replaced by 'housekeeper'.[9] The matron's office remained; but Privy Council rules in the 1860s ensured that the incumbent would not have the independence she had possessed under the old lay management system.[10]

The authority of the medical superintendents in respect of the attendants was more qualified. Theoretically the doctors would have liked to be in a position of unquestioned authority in matters of discipline and management. But while the superintendent could summarily suspend an attendant without having to provide a reason, the final decision on disciplinary action lay with the board of governors. Where the board failed to support the superintendent the latter's authority was diminished. Even without the complication of this two-headed structure, the physician might find disciplinary measures meeting subtle opposition from an attendant's colleagues, unorganised as this would be. The doctors were, of course, opposed to any form of organised unionism among their staff. When a National Union of Asylum Attendants in Ireland was formed in April 1896, with members at the Richmond asylum, it was swiftly dealt with by the superintendent (Conolly Norman) and the board of governors. Dr Norman warned of the dangers and disasters that would follow from an organised combination of this character; he was subsequently

empowered to dismiss two attendants who did not resign from the union following the governors' refusal to recognise it. At a meeting of the Irish branch of the Medico-Psychological Association (MPA) which discussed the union, most of the asylum doctors expressed confidence in their ability to prevent such an organisation getting into their asylums.[11] Direct challenges to their authority were rare. What was more difficult for the conscientious superintendent was actually knowing what his staff were doing, a problem which grew in magnitude as some asylums approached or passed a population of one thousand inmates.

The attendants were in daily intensive contact with the inmates to a degree approached by few asylum doctors. It was important therefore that their behaviour towards the lunatics be kept consistent with the aims of the institution. Ideally the superintendent would direct as much as possible the life of the asylum, the interaction between attendants and patients and between patients themselves. The asylum doctors highlighted the need for regulation in referring to their institutions in the language of technology. The governing principles of asylum care were outlined for attendants by the 1908 edition of the *Handbook for Attendants on the Insane*:

> An asylum is a complicated machine of many parts ... It is intended both by its structure and through its routine to be, in the first place, a house for the protection of the insane.[12]

It was a common metaphor for the asylum. A poor law medical officer in 1863 warned that from time to time suicides occurred

> even in the best regulated Asylums, with all their machinery of a large staff and separate system of wards.[13]

Similarly did John Nugent, the inspector of lunatics, refer to the 'costly machinery of an asylum' in 1874;[14] and the *Journal of Mental Science* in 1904 to the acquisition of land for St Patrick's Hospital in Dublin as the provision of 'a more efficient and economically curative machinery'.[15] To an observer of rare perspicacity like the English alienist John Arlidge, the machine analogy was adeptly used to criticise the very existence of the large public asylums in 1859.[16] It was a measure of the asylum's corruption from its original conception that, by 1908, this figure of speech could be used to epitomise the successful institution.

It was, of course, one thing to expect that the asylum would function with the routine and order of a machine and quite another to ensure that the structure of the machine was efficient to its task. Could a medical superintendent be confident that his attendants possessed the degree of tolerance, patience and self-control which the system of non-restraint, adopted after the 1840s, demanded? Would the asylum staff be capable of imparting those virtues which moral treatment implied, or of distracting the insane from their morbid preoccupations by engaging them in work, recreation, education and so on? These were major problems for asylum superintendents committed to creating 'hospitals for the insane'. And when they looked at the material they had to work with they were generally none too happy. For one thing there were still limits on the doctors' authority as far as appointments of staff went. Oscar Woods, medical superintendent of the Cork asylum, still found it necessary in 1887 to object to the appointment of staff by governors, claiming that it was the responsibility of the superintendent. It was a situation which, forty years before, John Conolly had described as 'extremely absurd'. For Woods, the competence of asylum staff in Ireland was seriously compromised by their coming from the same 'rank' as the patients.

> How much more control would they have over them if they were selected from a rank in life better educated, with feelings more refined, hearts more sympathetic?[17]

The class origins of attendants had not always been considered disadvantageous. Inspectors Nugent and Hatchell were struck 'with the kindly and familiar relationship existing in Irish asylums between their inmates, lunatics and servants alike'—this was attributed by them to the similar social origins of the lunatics and attendants (significantly equated in this passage as 'inmates'). Of course the two views are not necessarily inconsistent—kindly relationships alone would not inevitably conform with the principles and ends of moral treatment. And the inspectors themselves frequently expressed their concern at the rapid turnover of staff which disrupted the good order of the asylum. In 1863 they claimed that attendants frequently took employment with the sole object of earning a few pounds with which to emigrate.[18] Whether for this or other reasons there were constant changes in the staff most closely connected with the inmates. Reporting in 1883 that this was also a common problem in England and Scotland the inspectors noted that there had been a turnover of

128 in the average staff of 960 in Irish asylums in the previous year.[19]

The reasons for the high turnover of attendants were readily at hand in their wages and the conditions of work. Apart from security of employment there was little that was ostensibly attractive about a job that was sometimes dangerous and many times unpleasant. Wages were low, though reported as more liberal in some asylums such as Ballinasloe, Belfast, Clonmel and Richmond in 1865; at the bottom level in that year assistant male attendants were paid from £7 to £10 plus keep per annum (females £4 to £6).[20] In 1873 the attendants, lobbying for an improvement in conditions to the English level, claimed that the average wage of the 413 male attendants was 6s 9d per week, of the 443 females, 3s 9d.[21] These wages should be compared with those for agricultural labourers reported by the poor law inspectors in 1870—£8 to £12 per annum (£5 to £6 in Donegal and Derry) or 5s to 10s per week, depending on provision of food and lodging.[22] A compensating factor for asylum workers was that they received full board and clothing, in itself a reflection of their institutionalised status, since they also lived on the asylum premises; it is not surprising then that the inspectors of lunatics had once referred to the 'inmates, lunatics and servants alike'. Working hours were excessively long although, Inspector Courtenay claimed in 1910, the duties involved little actual labour but were sometimes dangerous and 'frequently call for the exercise of great forebearance'. He admitted that five asylums had average working days of thirteen hours or more and considered that the average weekly rates in Ireland were 82½ hours for day attendants and 75 hours for night attendants. The Waterford attendants who worked some of the longest hours claimed in a petition that a long day's duty could run to sixteen hours; they were allowed 2¼ hours off duty every second evening and every third Sunday off. In any struggle for better conditions the asylum attendants were faced not only with the opposition of the asylum management, which resisted higher wages and restricted working hours, but also with that of the doctors. The latter regarded restrictions on working hours as an attempt to limit the time 'that a person may devote to the interests of their patients'.[23] Although it seems there was little trouble in filling vacancies on the asylum staff the conditions of work were not likely to encourage stability in the establishment.[24]

In maintaining the routine of the asylum, medical superintendents were constrained not only by the high turnover of staff and the allegedly poor character of the recruits; a major problem as they saw it was the lack of training for the task. Sporadic attempts to instruct

attendants were evident from the late 1840s and no doubt an informal training in the control and management of the inmates was inevitable. At the Richmond asylum arrangements were made in 1845 'to allow a certain number of candidates [for positions of keeper or nurse] ... to attend at the asylum to receive the necessary instructions, in order to qualify them for the duties'.[25] In 1846 Francis White, the inspector of lunatics, recommended for the position of matron one of several women who had been attending at the Richmond asylum to qualify themselves for this office. He preferred these women over the several applications from matrons of gaols because 'much kindness as well as firmness of temper' are required in an asylum, implying 'a special training for itself alone'.[26]

Yet it appears that sustained and comprehensive attempts to train attendants especially for asylum work were not introduced until the 1880s when the alienists decided they wanted better staff. In an address which persuaded the MPA to institute special training for attendants, the Glasgow (Bothwell) asylum superintendent, Dr Campbell Clark, referred to the great aims suggested by Dr Clouston seven years earlier:

> To get the best raw material possible, and to manufacture out of it the best asylum attendant possible.[27]

The association decided to prepare an attendants' handbook and later instituted a certificate of proficiency in 'mental nursing'. In the 1890s Irish superintendents encouraged their attendants to undertake the study of the handbook, and themselves gave instruction in the elements of their 'profession'. Conolly Norman at the Richmond asylum gave some impetus to the training movement by making attendants pass an examination given by a member of the MPA as a test of promotion.[28] By promoting the training of these attendants the doctors served notice of their intention to 'hospitalise' the asylums. The move was not unchallenged nor always respected outside the asylums and there was considerable difficulty in establishing equality of status between general nursing and mental nursing. Only some consistent lobbying on the part of the MPA (rather than the asylum nurses) ensured that the nurses were included in the provisions of the Nurses Registration Act in 1919—in the meantime they were excluded, for instance, from the College of Nursing founded in Britain in 1916.[29]

With the training movement came the first sustained effort to

routinise the management of the insane under a medical model. The doctors implicitly recognised the inadequacy of their own contact with the insane in the now monumental public asylums. By profession-alising their staffs they strengthened their own authority within the asylum. The *Handbook*, the first editors noted, was designed to 'aid attendants to carry out the orders of the physicians'. But just how far this training should go and what it was intended to accomplish were difficult questions. Thus a reviewer (in the *Journal of Mental Science*) of the first *Handbook* questioned whether some of the details of physiology were necessary to attendants.[30] Perhaps it was the same writer who, in the following year, commended an Australian medical author for omitting 'all description of the anatomy and physiology of the brain in a book intended for the use of attendants and nurses'.[31] Not all members of the MPA agreed with this viewpoint. Consequently, the later *Handbooks* expanded the sections on physio-logy and anatomy, giving the practical aspects of the attendant's work very minor consideration. The emphases in the training and examination for the nursing certificate took the same path, leading, in the view of a later writer, to 'the deviation or heresy which led to the mental nursing qualifications being so largely divorced from the nurse's real work'.[32] What the training implied, then, was not any essential change in the relationship between doctor, attendant and inmate but rather a new conception of that relationship and its context. Doctors, by turning attendants into nurses, were countering that tendency to a 'lack of medical spirit in asylums' against which Conolly Norman cautioned in 1894.[33]

Given these qualifications about what the training movement meant we can now consider what these *Handbooks* told attendants about their relationship to inmates. With all the certainty of nineteenth-century psychological thought the attendants were told that the brain is the organ of mind: 'all disordered mental manifestations have their origin in derangements of the brain'.[34] The certitude gave way to relativity when an attempt was made to define the special characteristics of the insane. Deranged brains could only be made known through the person's conversation and conduct by comparison with the 'generality of his fellow-men' and with himself as he was before he became insane. The mental condition of every person varied from time to time but

when the variations are such as to render the person unable to take proper care of himself, or to behave rationally towards his fellow-

creatures, they are regarded as morbid and the mental condition is considered unsound.[35]

From this perspective insanity was, in fact, characterised chiefly by social disabilities and consequently the emphasis of treatment was on the correction of behaviour. 'Delusions' were not to be ridiculed but ignored; 'misapprehensions which so commonly exist in the minds of the insane' were to be explained 'rationally', we must presume, since the *Handbook* left this to the attendant's intuition. The staff would try 'to lead the mind into a more healthy groove of action, to repress morbid acts or habits'.

> All those acts and habits which spring from the diseased mental condition, and which are therefore morbid and unnatural, should be repressed as far as possible and correct habits inculcated in their place.

Hence the attendants were instructed to rectify the insane habits of the patients—their destructiveness, uncleanliness, slovenliness in dress, disorderliness in eating, bad sexual habits.[36] While uncivilised acts were in this way explained physiologically, such reproval of the insane had, of course, a long tradition of moral chastisement behind it. As the Irish inspectors had counselled some decades earlier, the asylum had the important function of social improvement to fulfil. For many of the inmates, the asylum provided for the first time an education in 'habits of order and cleanliness', an improved diet and 'servants at all hours to administer to their personal wants'.[37] From such a position derived the emphasis, sometimes no more than an ideal, on constant vigilance on the part of attendants in scrutinising the behaviour of the insane.

All the persons in the charge of attendants were 'patients', requiring special care and management. In the ordinary wards, therefore, just as in the sick-room, efforts should be made to secure 'tranquillity, due quietude, and cheerfulness'.[38] Although the title of the *Handbook* was unchanged until the seventh edition of 1923, the fifth edition of 1908 medicalised the attendant's relationship to the patient by using the terms 'nurse' and 'attendant' as 'equivalent and interchangeable'.[39] To emphasise the point the new *Handbook* laid down its second general principle of asylum care (the first being that the asylum was a complicated machine):

an inmate is now called a *patient* instead of a *madman* or a *lunatic*,
as of old, because it is recognised that he is ill and needs treatment.
That idea of him must always be preserved.

The advantages of this ideology were self-evident:

the idea that a patient is ill is a far better reason to give him for his
detention than that he is too troublesome, dangerous, or foolish to
be abroad.

But if the inmates were ill and the attendants nurses, then was the
asylum a hospital? The doctors who prepared the 1908 edition
admitted that some might find the label inappropriate. Their defence
of the new nomenclature was rather laboured. Just as in any hospital,
ordinary remedies for physical illness were administered in the
asylum. But, in addition, 'true medicine of a moral nature is given in
plenty in the shape of advice and control, though it is difficult to weigh
up or measure'. Moreover, what was special about the asylum was its
'discipline and routine' which might

well be compared to the hygiene of an ordinary hospital. They tend
to keep in subjection excitement and disorder, which are as harmful
to the mental invalid as microbes are to a patient with a wound or
sores.[40]

This concern to establish the legitimacy of their medical practice
betrayed the early psychiatrists' own insecurity on the matter. The
instruction given to attendants about their duties in relation to patients
reflected the determination of the MPA to upgrade the profession by
translating the language of asylums into that of hospitals and the most
advanced sections of the profession. There was no guarantee that
practice would thereby be altered. Indeed the prescriptions of the
Handbook in its various editions differ little from those of John
Conolly writing in the 1840s. How they were put into practice and
how they were experienced by the inmates was another matter. But we
should conclude this consideration of the ideology of attendance on
the insane by noting the conflicts within it. One part of this ideology
stressed the attendant's careful attention to the behaviour and thought
of individual inmates with a view to the creation of an environment
specially adapted to individual cases. Yet at the same time the
attendants were to conform to the dictates of the institution—they

were to study and obey the elaborate rules of the asylum, that smoothly running machine characterised by discipline and routine. Insanity was a relative matter, they were told, and each person's state of mind had to be judged in relation to the 'generality' of his fellow-men and to his own past. Yet the morality of moral treatment was not relative but absolute—cleanliness, order, right habits, the expulsion of bad thoughts and the inculcation of right ones. Inevitably, it seemed in the later nineteenth century, the growing size of asylums and the increasing permanence of the 'chronics' meant the priority of institutional values and absolute standards of behaviour over individual treatment. In the following pages we see how the asylum inmates themselves experienced these tendencies.

Institutionalisation

In 1894 Conolly Norman, superintendent of the Richmond asylum, warned his colleagues of the dangers of their own institutionalisation through what he described as the wearing, depressing and monotonous existence of asylum life. It was advice which starkly demonstrated the pessimism with which he and some like him were facing the future of the asylum. What he said about the effect of institutional life on the doctors could equally apply to its effects on the inmates. In particular there were tendencies in asylum life that made 'for narrowness, gloominess and sullen self-asserting isolation'. Asylum officers were counselled to 'individually struggle to maintain clearness and width of view, detachment of mind, the dry light of the intellect'.[41] Asylums, Norman began to think, were not conducive to recovery, nor even to a tolerable existence for many of their inmates. It would be better for many patients to be outside, boarded out with sympathetic families. Among the disadvantages of asylums he noted in 1896 that in

> the huge asylums which have sprung up or are now springing up everywhere, individual treatment—the one thing likely to benefit our patients—becomes almost impossible.[42]

Norman, as superintendent of the country's largest asylum, was speaking with a good deal of authority, though his advocacy of 'boarding out' was unsuccessful in Ireland. The effects of institutional life were clear enough every day in his own asylum. The omniscient and omnipotent superintendent of asylum theory quite obviously

found it impossible to know the circumstances of more than a thousand inmates. But even the institution, when it had reached this size, lost control of its charges. When a Richmond doctor reviewed the register of long-stay female inmates in 1898 she had to rely on the information of a nurse who had been there thirty years to confirm the identity of many of them. Even so she was forced to conclude that some patients still on the hospital register were probably dead because they 'could not be found'; and thirty-two years after the event, it was discovered that it was really Anne M— who had died on 1 March 1866, not Mary M—, who appeared still to be alive.[43] We can understand, therefore, the special poignancy of the 'memorial to the unknown pauper lunatic' erected in 1883 at the Colney Hatch Asylum in London at the spot where nearly 2,700 inmates had been buried *in forma pauperis* from 1851 to 1873.[44] Institutionalisation could reach the stage where the authorities lost sight of those for whom the asylum was established. It was against this that Conolly Norman protested.

Not all his colleagues were as sensitive to the ill-effects of the asylum on inmates. Thus another doctor, reviewing the long-stay male inmates in 1898, found a 56-year-old former labourer who had been admitted in 1880 'quite rational'. But his account of their brief interchange expressed surprise at the man's attitude.

> He is discontented for being kept here so long and becomes a little irritable and cynical if one suggests that he ought to like being here as he is treated so well.[45]

In these few remaining records of the interaction of doctors and their long-stay patients, the 'chronic', the 'incurable', we find glimpses of the numbing effects of the total institution.[46] In their ward-rounds, reviewing the status of inmates, doctors would repeat time after time the same series of questions designed to test memory, elicit delusions or hallucinations, discover whether the patient had recognised his or her 'mental illness'. Occasionally such a routine would meet with resistance as inmates expressed their irritation with the interrogation. When, after eight years in the asylum, an old woman was asked why she came there she replied that she had told the doctor before and '[did] not see the necessity for telling [her] again'.[47] Asking why the inmate was confined was part of a strategy designed to uncover the continuing presence of delusions or 'unfounded' dislikes of or accusations against people in the outside world. The aim is well expressed in the tense of

Conolly Norman's observation on a patient in 1897—he is 'quiet and depressed but *will not* express any delusions'.[48]

As well as 'why' the inmate came to the asylum, the doctor wanted to know 'when' as well as what day and year it was 'now'. A former labourer, re-admitted in 1891, says he has been there about ten years in 1902 but answers the same when seen again in 1904 and 1906. He 'has no idea of time'. By 1914, at the age of 52, he is described as 'this old man'. His memory the doctor describes as defective as he cannot tell the date or the days of the week.[49] But what did time mean in the asylum which was arranged to eliminate it? Every day was the same as any other—even the superintendent of the asylum felt threatened by the institution's 'monotony'. A rare case recalls the date of commitment nine years before,[50] but for most the asylum has killed time. Asked how long she has been in the Richmond, an old woman who 'was' a twenty-year-old servant when admitted makes one of her few replies to the doctor's interrogation—'I am always here, I live here.'[51] She had been 'here ... her lifetime', answers another.[52] After so many years in the asylum time had disappeared; ten, twenty or thirty years were much the same in 'such a place as this hell on earth' as one woman described it.[53] For these people the world stopped when they entered the asylum. Their memories were usually of relatives, often of those who had put them in. Harriet F— recalls that her mother 'sent her here [thirty years before] because she was contrary and ran about wild'. For some time after committal her friends visited her but she had not seen any relatives for twenty-five years.[54] Cut off from time and the outside world, how were the remaining years of life in the asylum experienced by these inmates?

While some looked forward to their death to the extent of already claiming to have experienced it, it was possible to find those who displayed some desire to go outside once again. After thirty-eight years, one man tells the doctor he has been in too long, and that a couple of years is long enough for anyone—he wanted to go out to work but when the doctor says he is too old he accepts the inevitability with 'I suppose so'. Four years later 'he is still very melancholic looking and sits in his chair with his arms folded and head bent down and eyes shut'.[55] The logic of the inmates' dependence on the institution was also brought to bear on Mary B—; asked, like the others, whether she is 'happy here' she says she is not 'because she will never get out'. But, adds the doctor's report, she 'has not the slightest idea what she would do if she did get out'. The report observes that she 'keeps her head bent down and hunches up her

knees'.[56] John Blake, the 1860s campaigner for 'moral treatment' in Irish asylums, considered that one of the admirable features of a good asylum, such as the Leicester institution which he had visited, was that there was little desire on the part of the inmates to get out. In nearly every Irish asylum he had visited he received numerous appeals to procure the liberty of an inmate.[57] Yet, whether or not an asylum was 'bad' or 'good', those who stayed more than two or three years were probably less likely to be in a position to demand their liberty, or even to take it when offered. A long-stay inmate told the Richmond staff in 1899 that he liked being there and would not want to leave—after nine years in the asylum, he had been discharged in 1876 but for some reason 'never went'.[58] Outside there might be only the less attractive resort of the workhouse—inside was a familiar environment and routine sustenance and, for many of these incurables, employment in the gardens or one of the asylum workshops. One ground of opposition to the establishment of auxiliary asylums for 'chronics' and 'incurables' was that these people frequently formed a substantial part of the asylum's workforce.[59] Thus a symbiotic relationship of inmate and institution developed, sustaining the life of both. Even where relatives might be expected to accept a discharged inmate the asylum could encounter considerable resistance. The inmates had to experience not only their own institutionalisation but their uselessness to those outside. Having received a request from the Omagh superintendent to take back an inmate the relative concerned replied that there was

> no one willing to take Noble into their home he is a great bother to the neighbours for he always gets worse when he comes home and would run about from place to place. It is better to let him die in the Asylum. Please send us word if he dies and we will pay expenses and bring him home. I was down about a week or two ago to see him.[60]

Those who died in the asylum had frequently spent a substantial part of their lives there. Their lives had become identified with it. But there were also those whose only experience of the asylum was as a place for the dying; or those whose probable future outside the asylum was cut short by disease contracted in it. This was a depressing reality for asylum authorities for whom the institution existed to promote the health of those who entered it. Doubtless it was behind the little-disguised antagonism of superintendents like Conolly Norman towards

the large institutions they were forced to work in. There was nothing the asylum could do for those who were admitted to the asylum in advanced stages of fatal illness. By the turn of the century, for instance, general paralysis was becoming a common cause of death among the male admissions to the Richmond asylum (and the asylums of other cities in Ireland). Doctors usually identified the disease quickly and death could come within a couple of months and certainly within a few years.[61] Another common cause of death among recent admissions was tuberculosis of the lungs. This was the case, for example, of Mary F—, a nineteen-year-old servant who died of phthisis, just twelve days after her committal from the South Dublin workhouse. In such cases the asylum existed to house the allegedly intractable rather than to treat in any sense—hence another such woman had been admitted from the workhouse which had its own infirmary but found it more convenient to pass on the troublesome sick to the asylum.[62] For yet another group of patients conditions in the asylum were directly responsible for their deaths. Every year the inspectors found it necessary to list asylums in which epidemics of typhus or dysentery had occurred during the year. Inevitably these took a toll of those who were already weak and debilitated on entering the asylum: thus James R—, of 'low bodily health' on admission, died within nine weeks from dysentery; Mary G—, 58, suffering from 'debility', and Mary R—, 18, recently discharged from the Hardwicke Hospital following an attack of pneumonia, were among the number who died during a dysentery epidemic in the Richmond asylum in November 1891.[63] By the turn of the century asylum authorities were being forced to look critically at the health standards of their institutions—tuberculosis and dysentery had become a serious threat to the lives of the inmates and even staff. Hence institutionalisation had two aspects. The dull, inertia-like surroundings of the asylum ('unhealthy' as Conolly Norman described them) would almost certainly foster 'dementia' where it was not already present; and the physically insanitary conditions nurtured disease and sometimes caused death. It was intolerable, thought the *Journal of Mental Science*, 'for a conscientious superintendent to think that patients suffering from mental disorder may come in for cure, but may be injured or killed by the evils of the establishment where they seek health'. Intolerable or not, such was the fate of too many who entered the asylum as the century approached its end.[64]

Treating the Curable: the Moral Agents

The lunatic asylums which had promised so much in the 1840s and
1850s were clearly less benign by the 1890s. But even at their worst
moments they were hosts to another population besides the dying and
the institutionalised. Always there were those whose stay in the
asylum was relatively short, ranging from a few days to some months.
They emerged in the asylum statistics as those discharged 'recovered'
or sometimes only 'relieved'. Some of them, of course, would return to
the asylum sooner or later but there were others who only once saw
the inside of an asylum. For both groups the asylum had a different
meaning, or at least was the context of a different experience, from
that of those whose lives had become inseparable from the institution.

It was by no means clear that the lunatic asylum had an *active* role
to play in the treatment of those whom it considered curable. Rather it
was to be the *context* of a readjustment of the patient's social and
mental world which might lead him or her back to good thoughts and
correct actions. The emphasis was on the construction of a favourable
environment within which a remission could take place—thus the
importance, as we have seen, of the omnipotent superintendent and
disciplined, well-trained staff. What exactly was effective in the
asylum's armoury was never made too explicit. But just as children
could only be brought up in a favourable domestic environment so
lunatics could only be mended in one. 'A lunatic asylum is a large
home' proclaimed the *Journal for Mental Science* in 1858.[65] By
providing an ideal home in place of one which presumably failed,
doctors might encourage a regeneration of their patients' mental
states. An Irish essayist who won the Lord Chancellor's prize for a
paper on insanity in 1847 insisted on the early and absolute
separation of the lunatic from friends and relatives and their removal
to an asylum 'where a new train of ideas will arise, and all former
associations be removed from his mind as much as possible'.[66]

The psychological school remained persuasive, though not necessarily
always dominant. An English psychiatrist in 1909 stressed the
importance of what he called 'psychic treatment'—staff should ignore
the patient's faulty ideas and attempt to build up in his 'reasoning
mind' a self-reliance and a moral conscience. The 'mental atmosphere'
of the ward was important—to encourage the patients that something
was being done to cure them inspired their confidence in both the
physician and the nurses and suggested to them that this was a time of
rest and relief from care and worry.[67] With the advent of 'psychotherapy'

in the Edwardian period the psychiatrists discovered that they had all along been practising its principles, or rather, what they thought were its principles. Dr Nolan of the Downpatrick asylum insisted that 'psychotherapy' was just a new phraseology to describe the old methods which most alienists had adopted: at the Limerick asylum, he recalled, Dr Courtenay had spent his whole morning walking the wards 'interviewing patients and ascertaining everything he could in connection with them. Next morning he went back to them, speaking to them in the manner which he found helpful in each case.'[68] This 'moral treatment' was empirical and intuitive. It was also, as Conolly Norman had pointed out, quite impossible in the large asylums.

For others the effective agent in asylum treatment was physical, the nourishment of the body and the elimination of any evident physical disease. Even for the psychological and moral treatment school, this was of course the *sine qua non* of recovery from insanity. But there were those, particularly in the 1870s and 1880s when the physical basis of mental illness was considered incontrovertible, who held a sanitorium view of the asylum. The president of the MPA in 1872 (Sir James Coxe, also a Scottish lunacy commissioner) claimed that there was nothing special about the treatment of insanity beyond adherence to the broad rules of hygiene. For him insanity was mainly the result of a deteriorated body, rather than a troubled nervous system. So the 'great secret' of successful treatment lay in

> supplying abundance of food and clothing, in providing a comfortable lodging and bed, in giving proper attention to cleanliness, and in affording ample means of varied occupation and exercise in the open air.[69]

Yet he himself was pessimistic as to whether asylums did or could provide this healthy environment: an asylum 'in itself' possessed no special virtue beyond 'the power of control which it confers, and the isolation which it facilitates'.[70]

Coxe's views, oriented towards the alleviation of the physical condition by provision of material comforts, represented one side of the 'physical' approach. The other was the search for a pharmaceutical panacea, a 'specific' for insanity. The use of drugs was ambiguous in motivation. Some were the means of physical restraint of a new sort, viz. chemical, and their use for this purpose was common and popular in the 1870s and 1880s though frowned upon by the turn of the century. Other drugs, their administrators claimed, would positively

contribute to the recovery of patients. Inevitably there was only a fine
line between such distinctions. Thus a 1905 review of the sedatives
and narcotics used in the treatment of the insane agreed with the
contemporary opposition to 'drugging' but advocated the use of a
depressant in cases of 'moral insanity':

> Such patients, when found to be getting out of hand and kicking
> against the rigid discipline of asylum life, are benefited considerably
> by a short course of hyoscyamus.

These cases were always female in his experience and the drug
transformed a 'termagant into a useful and obliging patient'.[71] But,
while drugs for the maintenance of asylum discipline had been
discovered, there was little optimism in the search for what Daniel
Hack Tuke, the prominent English alienist, called an 'anti-psychosis'.[72]

The object of asylum treatment was the alteration of states of mind
and the production, in particular, of socially tolerable habits and
behaviour. The means by which this was to be accomplished were, on
the above evidence, haphazard, empirical, and not founded on any
consistent theory of what was at the root of insanity. In practice the
success of 'treatment' was unpredictable and an inmate's 'recovery'
was frequently inexplicable. How then did inmates experience this
panoply of methods and attitudes which confronted them in the
asylum?

In their role as agents of moral treatment alienists walked the wards
talking to attendants and patients, occasionally spending some time
with a particular case, now and again (as the regulations demanded—
frequently at first, annually after the first year) noting conversations
and general progress in the case-books. We do not have evidence of a
dialogue between attendants and patients though this must have taken
place at an informal level; and attendants rather than doctors were
commonly in the position of knowing the accessible details of an
inmate's history and current state. As we have suggested above, it was
the nurses of the Richmond who provided much of the information,
even down to personal identity, on the long-stay inmates of the 1890s.
Before the discharge of a Cork lunatic in 1873, the attendant who was
immediately in care of him was minutely examined as to his
behaviour.[73] But otherwise we are left ignorant of what kind of
relationship (other than that of control, which is well documented and
examined below) and understanding existed between inmate and
attendant.

Between doctor and patient there was an uneasy relationship, frequently paternal, sometimes affectionate and kindly, in other cases barely disguising disgust. From many doctors there was certainly a good deal of sympathy, perhaps from some even a degree of empathy. But the dialogue between the doctor and the asylum inmate, where it existed, was frequently a dialogue of the deaf. If inmates became irritated at the barrage of questions about the date and cause of committal, doctors could be equally frustrated by what was for them the inaccessible language of the insane. When awake, a doctor noted of a young woman in the Richmond, she

> never saw anything worse than herself. Says that her own ghost frightens her more than anything. I cannot find out what she means by this.

In the course of another conversation some six months later she recounts her history being brought up as an orphan in the workhouse, sent to prison at the age of sixteen; about the prison 'she had various delusions and hallucinations which she recognised as such':

> But she says she was very much frightened in the prison by seeing three nuns on a step-ladder beating their foreheads with stones. And she will not allow that this is a hallucination. Says that when bad in her mind she believes herself to be dead ...[74]

While there were some things which had meanings obscure to the doctor, there were other statements, delusions and hallucinations, which the alienist considered himself especially qualified to recognise and eliminate if possible.

Sometimes such phenomena are played with in an attempt to demonstrate their absurdity. Mary C—, a 'noisy and troublesome' patient, demands to be let out after six years because she owns the world; she is the Blessed Virgin and must get out to her son Jesus Christ. The doctor teases her:

> surely such a person could leave this place whether we wished to keep her or no. She answered quite non-pulsed [*sic*]. How can I go when you lock the doors on me. I am kept here by the arch-anti-Christ Cullinan [one of the doctors] ...[75]

When Conolly Norman talks in 1896 to another woman who has been

in four years she declares that she was very bad in her mind when she came there but is quite well now. Nevertheless, he is not satisfied with her state of mind because she does not know 'the date of year' of her admission.

> She says it is four years ago. She accepts the suggestion that she came here in the year 1872! and having adopted that date she will not let herself be shaken in it.[76]

While doctors played games with the patients to remove absurd ideas or establish the current state of mind and reinforce their own rationality, they could themselves be confronted with the ruses of an inmate. A 'noisy and excitable' young woman who was very reticent under questioning plays up to her role 'when asked if anything was the matter with her':

> she opened her eyes widely gazed vacantly around her and then whispered—Mad—She appeared to realise much better than she pretended her surroundings and what was going on around her, occasionally a half conscious smile passed over her face or if she saw the ridiculous side of some of the questions she was asked.[77]

In the face of the mocking behaviour of the young girl the doctor was thus forced to question the common sense of his own diagnostic strategy.

The other response to the deluded language of the insane was to confront it with rationality rather than pursue it to absurdity. The standard of recovery was the decline of delusions and hallucinations, the admission that the patient had held a false view of reality, that he or she had been suffering from a mental illness, the reason for committal. The recognition of illness and the legitimating of asylum treatment was expected of patients, and even of relatives where they objected to continued treatment. Hence a rather agitated Dr Courtenay, as superintendent of the Limerick asylum, requested the inspectors' sanction to the discharge of an inmate: the father of the girl concerned 'believes that his daughter was wrongly sent to the Asylum—cannot be made to understand that this is the proper place for her'.[78] In her review of the long-stay patients in 1898 Dr Fleury of the Richmond asylum was anxious, vainly so, to gain their own admission of their insanity. One woman she talks to 'had not a proper recognition of mental illness'.[79] To recognise one's illness was the first step on the

road to rationality and discharge. The patient 'is quite rational', we read of a man who was admitted two months previously, complaining about voices telling him to drown himself; he is now 'fully aware that these voices are the result of a disordered brain'.[80] Similarly, six days before his discharge, another is reported to be 'aware fully of how deranged his mind has been'.[81]

Where outright admission of one's mental illness was not demanded, the doctor might still require a denial of previous delusions and perhaps a penitential confession of past wrongs. Recognition of one's violence or sexual aberration was a signal sign of success in the course of this moral treatment. On 26 July 1888, a week after committal, George E— is reported as being 'improved in manner and general conduct; but he resents his being sent to an asylum, as he states he has had only a few hot words with his wife when he was in liquor and trouble'. A month later, however, he has thought it over and 'now expresses regret for his past conduct towards his wife, and promises amendment when discharged'.[82] On admission a 23-year-old youth 'confesses that he has from early youth masturbated very much'. Six weeks later when questioned about it he says he is not now masturbating, 'that he sees the evil of it'.[83] A man described as epileptic has no delusions or hallucinations but, the case note adds, 'is confused and indignant that he should have been sent to an asylum'. He is less confused a few days later but he still refuses to acknowledge his mental state—he is 'constantly repeating that he is all right, and demands to get home'.[84] Behind these reports lies a persistent theme: the constant struggle to establish the dominance of the medical analysis of one's language and behaviour. The poignant message of a man who has spent thirty-nine of his fifty-seven years in the Richmond is that ultimately only one style of language is acceptable inside the asylum. When he is discovered talking 'gibberish' he is asked what language it is. It is 'snowball' language, he tells the staff—'you took my language from me'.[85]

Besides the haphazard and moralistic approach of 'individual treatment', moral treatment boasted other weapons in the campaign for 'mental diversion from morbid currents of thought'.[86] These were oriented towards the construction of new states of mind by the influence of a favourable environment. The emphasis here was on the collective treatment of the insane. In some asylums this aspect of moral treatment involved a positive direction of new thoughts and inculcation of improving values through a system of education or an emphasis on the guidance of religion. More common in the theory of

moral treatment was the encouragement of activities which achieved their purpose negatively: work, particularly agricultural (though only for men), and the provision of recreations. Both of these would lead the mind away from its morbid patterns.

The importance of work was a persistent theme of asylum authorities' reports and any lack of suitable provision for occupation of the inmates was constantly remarked upon. 'Nothing can be more injurious to the insane themselves than idleness', the inspectors claimed in 1862.[87] Potentially this aspect of treatment coincided with the asylum's financial interests. The manager of the Limerick asylum had reported in 1845 that outdoor work had made a profit for the asylum and this, the inspector noted, was 'in addition to the benefit it confers by allowing the patients sufficient space for air, exercise and recreation'.[88] At about the same time Inspector White advised that the new asylum at Mullingar should have attached to it 'at least from 50 to 100 acres of ground, particularly as four-fifths of the inmates will consist of the agricultural classes'.[89] Sixty years later, setting the inmates to work in the fields was not deemed any the less important; the inspectors in 1909 stressed the reduction of costs and the addition to the 'health and happiness' of the inmates, in that order.[90] So the patients were set to work, more vigorously at some places than others—at Ballinasloe and Killarney in the 1850s the men worked from morning to night in the fields.[91] Whether outdoor work was conducive to 'recovery' or not could hardly be demonstrated since a condition of its application as therapy was a willingness on the part of the inmate to undertake it. Such a decision could, in part, be taken as a sign of improvement. In any case it can hardly have done harm and the extra diet for those involved was greater in quantity if not necessarily in quality or composition.

The fresh air which was considered so important in the restoration and maintenance of health was not as readily available to the other inmates. Some worked in the various asylum workshops or helped in the maintenance of the asylum buildings. The women were mainly set to sewing; but they were also part of the asylum's general labour force of cleaners and launderers and some helped in the kitchens. Work went on inside as it did outside the asylum. In the district asylums this work never seems to have been remunerated although the inspectors had suggested in 1848 that a portion of the net profits of work done in the asylums (mainly from the sale of manufactured cloth which in 1847-8 had amounted to £3,629) be set aside to provide a temporary support for the discharged inmates.[92] It was those who had committed

crimes who had some justice shown to them in this respect. After 1893 the prisoners at the Dundrum criminal asylum were paid 'gratuities' on discharge for work done in the asylum: ten years before the governor had complained that it was difficult to get the patients to work since they were not rewarded for it (as they were at Broadmoor in England).[93]

Work was not always regarded as an agent directly therapeutic in itself. Rather the ability to undertake it was a sign of pending recovery, or at the very least a means of breaking the monotony of asylum life. After four days in the Richmond, Michael M—, who had been there before, requested to be sent to the farm. Three weeks after admission, another is reported to be anxious to get out to work in the wards and on the farm; so too is John F— who requests work after only two weeks.[94] But an asylum being what it was nobody could be forced to work. It was one of the means by which Inspector Nugent thought a lunatic institution could be 'divested' of the appearance of 'being simply the receptacle of lunatics or mad people'.[95] Yet that was what they were and there were many like the 26-year-old labourer in the Richmond in 1889 who spent his days 'crying and moaning', constantly drugged; he could not be 'induced' to work at any stage of his six months' residence.[96]

Where the therapeutics of work were ineffective recreation could be instituted. Again, the provision of facilities for recreation was part of the asylum's orthodoxy. But where some useful and economic purpose could be found for work, the institutional benefits of recreation were obscure and only the most enthusiastic asylum manager could maintain more than a token programme. Asked by a royal commissioner about the facilities for recreation at the Richmond in 1856, the lay manager, Samuel Wrigley, reported that the male patients played ball and some played draughts although nearly all the boards were gone; while the women danced once a week, read books, attended the school or played cards. Of two ball-courts for the patients, one was occupied by the apothecary's pigs. The asylum physician said there was insufficient provision for 'intellectual and pleasurable amusements' by which he meant a billiard table, back-gammon, an evening school and unspecified means of light recreation.[97] Robert Harrison, the visiting physician of the Dundrum asylum, agreed that there was little to occupy the minds of the patients—he had often regretted the want of such things:

a reading-room, or a room with pictures to excite or engage that

attention, so as to keep them from a gloomy mood, into which they fall when unoccupied on a wet day.[98]

At Cork the inspectors discovered bagatelle-tables and card-playing, 'than which latter', they thought, 'there is seemingly nothing more to the taste of an Irish lunatic'.[99] Recreation, as these attitudes show, was intended to counteract the depressing and tedious influence of asylum life rather than to be a positive therapy in itself. Where it was conceived of as an element of 'curative' treatment rather more determined efforts were made to revive the spirits of the inmates. At Belfast, it was reported, one method of recreation was a walk in the suburbs and country of up to 150 patients at a time 'accompanied by their own brass band'. This was regarded as having an excellent moral and curative effect 'by thus confiding in [the patients'] steadiness and correct demeanour'.[100] Institutional demonstrations of this style showed the outside world that the asylum had restored order, decorum and obedience in those who were previously uncontrollable. The visitors (aldermen of the city and their wives) who attended a ball for 300 inmates at the Richmond in 1862 were reported to be 'much struck, not only with the admirable order which prevailed, but with the docility and cheerful readiness with which the patients complied with the directions given them'.[101] Similarly, the *Belfast Newsletter* concluded its report of a 'soiree' at the asylum with a commendation of the patients for their conduct which was characterised by 'the strictest propriety and decorum in every respect'.[102]

Associated with recreation in moral treatment was education. This was, it is true, more commonly a part of the treatment of idiocy, an area in which real advances were being made in France but virtually ignored in Ireland. Yet there were some (particularly those who found it difficult to see that insanity was anything more than a disorder of intellect) who thought that education had a role to play in the asylum, both by diverting the mind from its preoccupations and by exercising it. A particularly enthusiastic, even fanatical, advocate of an education system for asylums was Joseph Lalor, superintendent of the Richmond asylum from 1857 to 1883. As with all aspects of moral treatment, the efficacy of education of the insane was not very clear but its functional nature was never doubted by its supporters. Lalor found it a 'powerful, improving and ameliorating agent with all classes of the insane' but warned his audience in 1878 that its curative results might take years. He employed a number of 'trained' schoolteachers as officers, and organised the daily routine of inmates round periods of work,

educational instruction and recreation.[103] Daniel Hack Tuke and
other members of the MPA visited the asylum in 1875 and found the
system of some interest.[104] But there is no evidence that it was adopted
on the same scale elsewhere in Ireland or that its alleged therapeutic
qualities were anything more than the alleviation of institutional
monotony. For John Fox, the Richmond schoolmaster, the 'School
System' afforded 'intellectual food' to the minds of the insane and was
admirably calculated to heal the disordered faculties of those who
might be restored to society. However, from his review of the system it
was clear that the most it could have accomplished was the provision
of another means of occupation for the ever increasing number of
inmates.[105]

If the re-direction of the intellectual faculties was an important
prerequisite for recovery from insanity, the inculcation of correct
moral values was indispensable. For most doctors this meant some
role for religious intervention in the asylum. But what this role was to
be and who was to impart the appropriate values was a matter of
dispute. The relation of religion to the practice of psychological
medicine was ambiguous. In evidence given to the royal commission
on Irish asylums in 1856 few doctors contested in any way the value
of religious services in the asylum. But, for alienists, the value of
religion to an individual inmate was frequently tempered by the
latter's capacity to appreciate its virtues and truths. We have touched
on the important dispute centred on the appointment of asylum
chaplains at Belfast in another context. But in concluding our
overview of the day-to-day practice of moral treatment we must
consider the place of religion in the asylum's therapeutics.

For Robert Harrison, the Dundrum physician whose woolly ideas
about recreation we have already noted, moral treatment was in fact
educational instruction and recreation.[103] Daniel Hack Tuke and
question about the means of moral treatment at Dundrum:

> They speak to their people and advise them, and lecture them
> quietly and gently. There is no religious controversy, or anything of
> that kind—mere moral advice.[106]

But few doctors after the 1850s would have been as comfortable as
this about the place of institutional religion in their asylums. John
Conolly had warned physicians of 'the danger of misapplying
religious attentions'. The problem was, as he noted, and many others
after him, that 'no cause of mania, melancholia, and imbecility is more

common than a gloomy religion'.[107] In any asylum there were many whose prominent symptoms were of a religious nature—those like Anne M— in the Richmond who said religion had upset her mind, or Mary M— who thought her soul was lost and that she had not prayed enough.[108] And in Ireland there were sensitive sectarian issues involved which could also excite the minds of asylum inmates. A 26-year-old Catholic in the Richmond complained of his being tormented by everyone, people telling him one day he was a Catholic, the next a Protestant; on admission, a Protestant poured forth tirades against the papacy and said that his religion caused him to be subjected to the greatest cruelties.[109]

The rawness of the religious question in Belfast was unquestionable and in the 1850s and 1860s the governors of that asylum and the resident physician steadfastly opposed the government's attempt to appoint chaplains, arguing that they would be a divisive influence in the asylum. Over-zealous pastors might disseminate 'a wild and dangerous fanaticism amongst lunatics', disturbing the asylum's 'comfort and tranquillity'. Furthermore, the objection to the clergyman was that he was unable to judge the state of the patient's receptivity to religious values, something, it was claimed by the defenders of the Belfast system, which the resident physician alone could do.[110] In conformity with this view it was Dr Stewart, not the chaplains, who conducted the religious services in Belfast. The inspectors argued against the Belfast attitude (shared at Armagh, where appointed chaplains were also absent) claiming that religion, properly imparted by the official chaplains, could act as a 'sanatory agent' and that the fears of sectarian strife were unfounded in a public institution 'fenced in as it is with all the safeguards which an efficient staff and perfect discipline insure'.[111] Eventually the government legislated to force the governors to appoint chaplains of the major denominations.

These teething troubles in establishing the place of religion in the asylum were not experienced in most other Irish asylums. In the institutions in the south and west the religious composition of the asylum populations was overwhelmingly Catholic. It would have been politically uncomfortable for superintendents, frequently Protestant before the end of the century, to have opposed the active participation of the chaplains. But the doctors did agree with the Belfast superintendent that they should have the power to restrict the access of anybody, chaplains or relatives, to one of their patients. And this principle was enshrined in the conditions under which chaplains were appointed. The Privy Council rules and regulations required that

chaplains not infringe the medical barriers erected round the inmates by superintendents. When a Wesleyan minister in Maryborough protested that he had been refused permission to visit the asylum the Under-Secretary informed him that he could only visit Wesleyan patients and at 'such times as may be deemed not medically objectionable'.[112]

Moral treatment—through the agency of work, recreation, education or religion—and its less articulated but none the less practised companion, 'individual treatment' through a rational therapy, attempted to create a controlled environment directing the inmate towards habits and values which would conform to those of the outside world. However, the degree of its efficacy was always unknown. The therapeutic relationship between the asylum and its inmates was shrouded in uncertainty and the suspicion that recovery could just as well be spontaneous. When a Richmond doctor passively noted that a patient 'gradually lost all his delusions, and has taken a rational view of his present position and future prospects',[113] he was acknowledging the apparent uselessness of his own role in the transition. In this context moral treatment reflected the need to establish a system which, while maintaining routine and discipline, would make the asylum something other than a prison or a workhouse. To the extent that any asylum did this the authorities could be satisfied with a judgement of the *Freeman's Journal* that a day of athletic games and a night of dancing at the Richmond asylum had shown 'the progress of intelligence and the consequent advancement of Christian refinement and kindly sympathy with the stricken, the defenceless, and the afflicted'.[114] Yet the doctors were not content with the implication that they were merely agents of an improved system of good works. For them the indispensable sign of all that was special about nineteenth-century lunatic asylums was that they practised medicine in them.

The Physical Agents

Whatever school of thought predominated at any one time in the world of psychological medicine there were few who denied that the treatment of the insane involved physical treatment. The good alienist of the 1860s was a physician with a knowledge of mind, as James Crichton Browne put it; the great advance in psychological medicine had been when 'morbid conditions of the mind' were recognised as dependent on disease of the body and thus handed over to the medical

profession.[115] But as to practice we may note that the range of medical treatment in the asylum reflected the physician's uncertainty about what he was supposed to be restoring and how the agents he used acted on it. As always we need also to remember that the physician was superintendent of a large institution and responsible for maintaining its order. The methods of treatment adopted were commonly in danger of becoming punishment or of simply maintaining the peace by any means possible.

With so many admissions in a 'low state of bodily health' an obvious priority was physical restoration. This meant in some cases treatment in the asylum hospital for recovery from the effects of violence[116] or disease of one kind or another; for most admissions it meant a regular diet, if a spartan one, and for some a special diet to assist their recuperation from a heavy bout of drinking. Those like Joseph M— or Christopher K—, both of whom were received into the Richmond after a reported fortnight's drinking without food, were subject immediately to restorative diet and tonics.[117] On admission Francis G— appeared quite sane but had evidently been drinking hard; with 'dietic [*sic*] and tonic treatment' and a drug to help him sleep, his tremor diminished within two days and he was discharged a week later.[118]

It is difficult to judge how well the general asylum population was fed. The amount *per capita* spent on 'provision' varied enormously from one asylum to another—from £7 in Sligo to £13 in Dublin in 1871 and in 1910-11 from £6 13s in Downpatrick to nearly £11 in Clonmel—but these differences were determined partly by variations in local agricultural prices and probably significantly by the extent to which the asylum provided for its own needs.[119] There was no doubt, however, that asylum inmates were fed better than those of workhouses and, at least early in the period, of gaols. In 1868 a government committee noted that the workhouse diet for some classes of inmates was only two meals a day; and the gaol diet of two meals had been reduced in 1849 following charges that it was better than a labourer's or a workhouse inmate's diet.[120] The asylum diet, on the other hand, was invariably three meals, monotonous as they might be—the dietary table at Armagh in 1856 was 2¼lbs of stirabout (a porridge, usually of oatmeal, occasionally with the addition of rice) plus milk for breakfast, ½lb of bread with soup or milk for dinner, and the same amount of bread with milk for supper. The dietary tables, the report of the royal commission noted, showed some substantial differences from the returns of consumption for the same year. While the

Richmond dietary table indicated that half a pound of meat a day was allowed each patient, the stores return for the previous year showed an average per patient per day of less than one ounce. In general, the returns of consumption for 1856 indicated a diet of bread, oatmeal, rice, potatoes, meat (in the form of soup) and milk with some use of tea and sugar.[121] The absence of vegetables from the dietaries of asylums (not even potatoes in some) led to outbreaks of scurvy at the Cork asylum in 1852 and at Maryborough in 1868. With the development of asylum farms this aspect of 'treatment' probably improved.[122]

A more remarkable feature of the Richmond diet for some years was the place of 'stimulants'. Besides liberal amounts of education, Dr Lalor was evidently giving some of his patients even more generous amounts of liquor. In Sligo only 333 pints of sherry wine were consumed in 1873 and in Cork the average consumption of beer and porter was 26·6 pints over the year; in the Richmond the 981 patients had consumed 108,395 pints of beer and porter as well as 1,765 pints of whisky and 2,803 pints of wine.[123] In a veiled reference to the wide variation in alcohol consumption the inspectors had suggested in 1857 that 'the class of patients generally belonging to the metropolis, and larger cities and towns, require a more tonic dietary than the inhabitants of purely agricultural districts'.[124] But the impact of temperance led to a readjustment of attitudes in the 1870s and 1880s. Although some superintendents resisted the move as the deprivation of a comfort which helped make the life of the inmates tolerable, the MPA encouraged the abolition of drink in the asylums.[125] The result in the case of the Richmond was a reduction in expenditure on wine, spirits and beer from £940 in 1872 to £363 in 1911 for more than three times as many inmates.

If we are to use the standards suggested by the 1868 committee the impression of asylum dietary is that it was of the level of a rural labourer's diet. But it did at least have the advantage of regularity when food outside the asylum was frequently short—in the early 1860s and at many times in the 1880s and 1890s, together with that period of uncertainty every year between the end of last year's crop and the new harvest. If we are looking at the cities the asylum diet was probably a good deal better than the slender sustenance of tea, bread, potatoes and bacon which was the staple of the poor in the Dublin tenements in 1906.[126] And compared with English asylum inmates Irish lunatics were possibly fed better (or at least in greater bulk). A review of dietary tables by an Irish asylum superintendent in 1886 concluded that approximately the same amount of meat was consumed

in Irish and English public asylums. Of the other foods consumed, the Irish inmates were reported as having substantially more bread, potatoes and milk and slightly more vegetables (the amount of the last seemed to depend on asylum production of them). The working inmates of the Irish institutions probably consumed the difference; non-working inmates were fed on large quantities of Indian meal and oatmeal.[127]

A good diet and the special provision of 'tonics and stimulants' was considered the most basic pre-condition of recovery: a healthy mind could only exist in a healthy body. But what of the doctor's other 'medical remedies'? We have already seen that the search for a panacea in the form of a drug was viewed with pessimism. But this is certainly far from implying that drugs had no place in the asylum. Rather their role was regarded as indispensable as the century progressed. At Armagh in 1846, for example, Dr Kidd considered that 'no individual medicine can be called particularly efficacious, much less specific, in the case of insanity'. The use of drugs was instead directed towards the maintenance of a *'corpus sanum'*, the limit of the medical contribution to restoring the *'mens sana'*. The physician at Clonmel was similarly sceptical, considering that it would be easier to give an opinion as to the *inefficiency* of medicines as a cure for insanity. Still there were those in the 1840s who insisted on the relevance of the traditional physical treatments. Thus Dr Rogan of the Derry asylum, while concentrating on the improvement of the general health by the use of tonics, diet and so on, also practised topical bleeding, blistering of the shaved head and nauseating doses of tartarised antimony in acute cases. But his list of recoveries suggested either that the physical method did not work or that it was only rarely applied—six cases recovered under medical treatment, fifty-six under moral treatment. Dr White of Carlow also practised some of the old methods, using bleeding and purgatives, but had also introduced the use of the drugs opium and hyoscyamus to procure 'composure and sleep'.[128] The extent to which these methods were practised in any asylum is obscure particularly as no records of prescription were kept in many institutions—at Cork between 1847 and 1853 prescriptions were made on the verbal directions given to the apothecary or attendant.[129] But in 1857 the inspectors could not say that any particular medical treatment for the cure of insanity was resorted to, 'except in its early stages'. The malady was little understood and 'air, regimen, exercise with the removal of causes leading to excitment' were regarded more favourably.[130]

However, throughout the 1860s and 1870s drugs were becoming a more attractive medical treatment. Asylum doctors were experimenting on their patients, sometimes even on themselves, in the search for sedatives and sleeping drugs which were efficient without producing obvious deleterious effects on inmates.[131] Still, the increasing use of drugs was accompanied by some disquiet at the motivation for and implications of the practice. Thus in 1877 Dr Lockhart Robertson, a prominent English alienist, had to defend the use of narcotics and sedatives in response to a question about 'chemical restraint' from a parliamentary committee.[132] Restraint, of course, was the motivation where there was a need to control violence: in an article on 'use and abuse of chloral hydrate', George Savage of the Bethlem Hospital warned of its ill-effects but suggested that 'it may be used rather as restraint than as treatment in violent cases'.[133] But there was no clear opposition between 'restraint' and 'treatment' in the management of many asylum patients, not just the violent. When S.J. Cullum summarised for readers of the *Dublin Journal of Medical Science* in 1905 the use of 'Sedatives and Narcotics in the Treatment of the Insane' his criteria were as much the maintenance of asylum discipline and order as the state of health of the patient. The sedative sulphonal was to be used with a class of patients 'which was one of the most troublesome in the asylum ward'; cannabis indica kept the patient, particularly the senile dement, 'quiet and manageable during the day'; as for epileptics—'the most troublesome and dangerous class ... found to be the cause of every disturbance in a dormitory'— the hypnotic, chloral hydrate, gave the best results for pacifying them, and the bromides not only lessened the fits but enabled the doctor to get the 'epileptic to work well'.[134] The conditions of life in large institutions had come to determine the criteria for administration of 'therapeutics', though not without regret or unease among doctors. The discussion after a paper on the use of hypnotic drugs in the treatment of insomnia disclosed considerable division of opinion over whether hypnotics should be administered as a 'restraint'. Charles Mercier, the London psychiatrist, took the hardheaded line that the patient was committed to be 'treated, detained and restrained'. Others were less comfortable about their role in the last of these responsibilities and the means chosen to go about it.[135]

The major problem with drugs was that they almost invariably had harmful physical consequences; the absence of clinical trials of a conclusive nature meant that asylum doctors discovered the ill-effects too late. As T.S. Clouston bluntly put it in 1883 when talking of the limits on medical treatment of 'senile insanity':

My experience of opium and herbane is unfavourable as sedatives; they diminish the appetite and often kill the patient.[136]

Cullum, in the article we have already discussed, openly acknowledged two cases in which he had administered drugs resulting in death.[137] A typical experience with a new drug was that of Conolly Norman. In November 1888 he delivered a paper to his Irish colleagues on a new hypnotic, 'Sulphonal', which he praised for its efficiency in procuring sleep. In the following years he administered it freely in the Richmond asylum, as did many others in Ireland and Great Britain following him. However, its success in the treatment of sleeplessness was complicated by its other effects in those, for instance, whom it made 'dizzy' or 'queer'.[138] Twelve years after he had introduced it he told a meeting of the MPA that he now considered it disadvantageous to the patient. In fact the drug was found to be accumulating in the kidneys causing poisoning and death after continued administration.[139] Thus, even where the administration of drugs was uncomplicated by the suspicion that it was merely a new form of restraint, doctors could find that their resort to physical remedies harmed the patient.[140]

Beyond drugs there was the occasional adoption of some other palliative for insanity. Some of these innovations promised much on their inception, no doubt through the change in the institutional environment which might accompany them. Thus in 1860 'Turkish baths' were constructed at some considerable cost in the Cork asylum. The resident physician was soon claiming a 76 per cent cure rate with the baths—what he meant was that 96 patients (of nearly 500) had been treated in this way in 1861 and 74 had been 'cured'. The bath was at least pleasant, even if, as the inspectors noted, no 'direct curative effects' could be attributed to it:

those who had suffered a relapse (the physician claimed) ... showed no unwillingness to return to the Asylum; and even asked to be taken there at once, in order that they might get the bath, as they considered that nothing else would cure them.[141]

Yet most physical treatments had less of this benign quality and in the way they were applied were a form of punishment. The most controversial example was the use of cold shower-baths or ordinary baths as a means of controlling or calming an inmate.

Most asylums in the 1850s had shower-baths which were to be used only under doctor's orders. The shower-bath was administered,

according to Harrington Tuke in 1858,

> for one of its three effects ... these are 'the shock', the 're-action', and the direct refrigerant or depressing effect produced by a continuance of the shower or its frequent repetition.[142]

Whether or not doctors had control of its use in everyday practice was uncertain in the Irish asylums. Samuel Wrigley, the Richmond manager, reported that there was a shower-bath in each division of the asylum and that one was being installed in each ward; he never knew an attendant to give one without orders. But the attendants had the keys; and Wrigley's other evidence showed that he infrequently visited the wards, so he was unlikely to know when it was used or not.[143] Robert Fitzgerald, the resident physician of the Limerick asylum, had never read the regulation requiring the instruments of restraint to be kept by him.[144] Although a therapeutic rationale had been constructed for the bath, shower-bath and douche (throwing buckets of cold water over the patient), by the 1870s it was commonly considered that they had come to be used 'solely for the maintenance of discipline'. Some superintendents therefore had stopped using them.[145] The state of affairs in asylums where these methods of control were used was highlighted at Limerick in 1872. There Dr Fitzgerald ordered a plunge-bath to be administered to an undisciplined patient—the attendant, using other patients to 'duck' the patient, had caused his death by submersion.[146] After this, although the Privy Council rules made the use of baths discretionary to the superintendents, most doctors deplored the practice. In 1887 Dr O'Farrell (then a medical inspector with the local government board) condemned the custom in Ennis workhouse of 'punishing' excitable lunatic patients with cold shower-baths—it was 'a relic of a barbarous age'.[147] Yet in the criminal asylum in Dundrum in the same year Dr Ashe was still defending the use of the plunge-bath as a means of punishing an inmate who had caused a disturbance in the chapel. Such use was still permissible under the rules. Despite this the Under-Secretary wanted to know what steps the inspectors of lunatics proposed to take 'to render the use of the bath as a punishment impossible'; he found, he told the Chief Secretary who was expecting parliamentary questions on the matter, 'that all Drs except apparently Dr Ashe condemn its use'. Shortly after, the government forbade its use as a punitive measure.[148]

The relative failure of physical (medical) treatment brings us back

to the relationship between doctor, attendant and patient. By 1883 the superintendent of a large London asylum could note that with the absence of medical appliances (he meant electrical apparatus and baths) and the declining use of sedatives it was easy to see why the drug and surgical instrument account in asylums generally averaged only ½d a week per head. There seemed 'little in the treatment of the insane nowadays ... beyond good dietary, open air occupations and protection'.[149] Doubtless it was from this scepticism with regard to the potential of conventional medical treatment that the asylum doctors looked to the training of their attendants in the 1880s and 1890s. But what could be done in this area was limited by the very size of asylums, which made it difficult to supervise the activities of the staff, and by the poor working conditions which allegedly limited the quality of the attendants employed and the demands which could be placed on them. The result was that the relationship between attendants and patients was characterised by custodial considerations which spilled over into violence. Indeed it was in the violence which could characterise social relations in the asylum, between attendant and inmate and between inmates themselves, that the illusion of the asylum as a healthy environment was fully displayed.

Custodial Care and Violence

Everyday life in the asylum was centred on the continual struggle to wrest some order out of the chaos which surrounded doctors and attendants. While the 'quiet and respectful', the 'tractable', could be easily managed on assignment to the various work duties, the 'troublesome' were a constant source of tension and conflict. Some lay on the floor, crying if they were taken up, or roaring and rolling about.[150] Others sported the evidence of having annoyed fellow-inmates. Sarah O—, a 27-year-old servant who spent a year in the Richmond before discharge, was frequently 'very refractory, running about the wards, stripping herself and throwing herself into the other patients' beds'; as a consequence she was seldom without a black eye.[151] The restlessness and agitation could easily be translated into violence between inmates. Only three days after admission a young labourer was knocked down by one patient in the grounds of the Richmond then struck on the head with a stone by another, fracturing his skull.[152] In 1873 Thomas Hopkins choked John Ray, a very popular inmate, to death in the Ballinasloe asylum. Subsequently

Hopkins was himself under continual threat from the other patients and was attacked by one of them; they would 'not even sit or eat at the same table' with him, reported the superintendent.[153] One night in July 1889, the patients in one of the female wards at the Richmond saw Alice Chapman kill Ellen Deegan with a chamberpot; it was half an hour or more before the night nurse discovered the event.[154] When one Castlebar inmate attempted to commit 'an unnatural offence' (sodomy) on another, he was assaulted by the latter and died four days after from what was diagnosed as peritonitis.[155]

Many patients required continual observation, to prevent not only such assaults but also suicide. All asylums had their 'suicidal' divisions and in some the suicidal patients were specially marked out by caution-cards issued to the attendants in charge of them. Nevertheless under-staffing and carelessness or indifference on the part of attendants meant that every year saw suicides or fatal 'accidents' in the asylums. At Ennis in 1894 Mary Nicholl was one morning being taken with the other patients for the weekly bath when she threw herself through a glass window and fell to her death.[156] When Michael Fitzpatrick died at Castlebar in 1898 after drinking some disinfecting fluid, the inspectors found that there was some negligence on the part of the head attendant who had not ensured that his subordinates attended to their duties instead of leaving 'so much to be done by patients'.[157] The watchfulness of attendants was frequently enjoined in the aftermath of such incidents. But even instructions for the special care of individuals could be carelessly administered. The Castlebar superintendent had especially warned his staff to take special care of one man; but when he was taken out with other working patients to fill a pond with stones he jumped into it and drowned.[158]

Further, the trying nature of the attendants' duties and of the environment in which they worked is reflected in the hostility directed towards them and the medical staff. 'When passing through 17 Division last evening', we read in a Richmond case note, 'patient G— attacked me whereupon Mary E— "just as the row was going" thought she might have a try also and if she could would have smashed me'.[159] Patients who had been quiet for long periods of time would unexpectedly attack the staff. John L— had been 'very quiet' in his mood for six months until he jumped up from dinner and struck Attendant Shore in the face; Dr Rambaut in the Richmond could remember himself being similarly attacked by this man five years before.[160] At the asylum in Derry in 1858 an inmate, John Kane, entered an office, bolted the door, then attacked one of the governors

with a knife, wounding him in the forehead and temple. A few months later Margaret Kelly of the Maryborough asylum assaulted Dr Jacob with a 'flagging-stone'. Inspector Nugent considered that lunatics in asylums were frequently not only difficult to manage but personally very violent 'cognizant as it were that they have a *privilege* to be so'.[161] Yet the control of this violence, the government's law advisers noted in 1875, was in some ways the *raison d'être* of asylums. The Ennis superintendent wanted to prosecute two inmates for 'violent and dangerous assaults' on two attendants; he also wished to have them transferred to Dundrum, if only as 'an example to the other inmates many of whom have strongly urged on me that the criminals should not be kept in the institution'. But the law officer objected that it would not be proper for the mere sake of *'discipline* or *convenience'* to apply the ordinary criminal law to such inmates. There were no legal objections to proceeding against a lunatic who committed a crime, but the offence should be more than the 'ordinary assaults' which 'the prison (that is the asylum) discipline should as a matter of routine provide for'. The Attorney-General agreed with him that a person committed as a dangerous lunatic should 'be subjected to proper control in the asylum to which he is consigned'.[162] In other words, the government's legal officers were advising, the function of a district asylum was to contain the violence within it and not expect this problem to be solved by the use of the special criminal asylum in Dublin.

In this context then, the attendants and medical staff had to accept the relative immunity of their charges from the norms of the world outside. The asylum was supposed to be a hospital but as well had to impose a 'prison discipline' to protect the lives of inmates and other staff. A balance between these two imperatives was the object of an ideal administration of the asylum. But, in practice, the relationship between attendants and inmates frequently dissolved into mutual fear and consequent violence. Conolly Norman was appalled by the succession of assaults on patients and the indiscipline of his staff in the 1890s. After an attendant had beaten Michael Sheridan in 1895, breaking a rib and bruising his legs, Norman warned the acting head attendant that the govenors were determined to 'leave nothing undone to put a stop to the practice of assaulting patients'.[163] But he had already found that he could not rely on the board of governors to support him in disciplining the staff, and that attempts to censure the attendants could be counter-productive. In 1894 the governors had dismissed two nurses who had assaulted a patient; but Norman had

later complained of insubordination of the nurses in the same ward which had become difficult to manage since the inquiry into the previous case. On this occasion the governors did not support his case for dismissal. In the interests of institutional order Norman concluded that suspension of staff was not in itself always advisable.[164]

Clearly the attendants were required to exercise a great degree of self-control in many situations and when they were disciplined or dismissed for violent actions their colleagues might resent it. In 1890 an attendant was dismissed by Norman after the death of O'Connor, a 'violent, restless and powerful' patient (himself formerly head attendant at Dundrum; he had developed general paralysis). The inspectors themselves regretted that alternative means of control, seclusion or even the 'preferable evil' of restraint, had not been sought to manage O'Connor—on one occasion he had been locked in a corridor alone with an attendant, 'a course involving necessarily constant struggles, and probably consequent passion, so that in the end it might become a trial of strength between the two men—whether the patient would overcome the attendant, or the attendant overcome the patient'.[165] Yet Norman was angered by the case and went to some trouble to find witnesses to the assaults on O'Connor. In doing so he was evidently antagonising the other staff. He had found some patients who witnessed the event but 'they say that they will not give any evidence while living here, as it would not be safe to do so. In the latter point, I have no doubt their statements are well grounded.'[166] The implications of a reign of terror by attendants against the patients and the lack of confidence in his staff were no doubt two weighty reasons behind Norman's disillusionment with asylums.

The impression gained from the number of assaults coming to the notice of Dublin Castle in the 1890s and after was that there had been a substantial worsening of relations in the asylums. The crucial factor was probably the overcrowding, combined with a bad staff/patient ratio: one head nurse at the Richmond complained that she had 180 patients in her charge in 1891, with six assistants to manage them. Staff/patient ratios varied from ward to ward according to the classification of patients: the more intractable the patients, the more staff required, in theory at least. Yet at all levels, the ratios had almost certainly worsened between the 1850s and the 1900s. In 1858 a number of asylums had ratios as low as one attendant to eight males or one to five females. By 1901 nearly all Irish asylums exceeded the inspectors' recommended levels of one attendant to eleven or twelve patients. The Richmond asylum was among the best.[167] Coincident

with overcrowding was the dramatic increase in the absolute size of asylums since the 1850s.[168] This made it even more difficult for the superintendent to know what was happening in the asylum and to exert discipline over the attendants. As well we should recall that alternative means of controlling the lunatic (that is alternative to direct personal control by the attendants) had been progressively reduced. In the 1880s there had been some return to the practice of mechanical restraint.[169] But in 1896 the inspectors of lunatics moved to tighten the regulations governing restraint since 'public opinion is in favour of reducing its use to a minimum'.[170] 'Chemical restraint' was also in some disfavour, as we have seen above, and drugs were possibly less used by the turn of the century than they had been in the 1870s. In this situation the opportunities for violent confrontation between attendant and patient probably increased. Moreover, there was a tendency on the part of some asylum authorities to take the side of the attendants before that of the inmates. After the inspectors had failed to procure the dismissal of an attendant from the Sligo asylum following his assault on a patient they informed the government that they had recently observed 'a tendency on the part of the Committees of some of the asylums to condone offences of this nature'.[171] The alternative procedure for the government was the prosecution of the offending attendants, a difficult course because of the controversy over the status of a lunatic's evidence.[172]

The depressing conclusion for those who looked carefully at the asylum system around 1900 was that the treatment of mental disease, if that was what the institutions were about, was profoundly retarded in relation to other branches of medicine. The inspectors feared, following the Sligo case mentioned above, that public asylums would soon not even have the respectability of being 'places of shelter' but would be viewed with 'dislike and dread'.[173] The physical amenities of Irish asylums may have been markedly in advance of those in the workhouse hospitals, as a government inquiry into the poor law in Ireland remarked in 1906.[174] But under that surface there was, Conolly Norman argued, something 'unhygienic in the moral atmosphere of large institutions'. If it was possible that some of the patients did not feel this as much as might be expected, he still had no doubt of his conclusion when he looked at the 'marked deterioration of disposition' in the nurses and attendants who were 'to a large degree the instruments by which we work upon our patients'.[175] Norman's pessimism related essentially to the experience of the permanent population of asylums. As if to demonstrate the irrelevance of the

nature of the institution to recovery, the 'cure-rates' in 1911 were much the same as they had been forty years earlier. Much the same proportion of admissions, one-third, was being discharged within one year; and in 1911 those discharged had spent much the same amount of time inside as in 1871, that is 80 per cent for less than one year.[176] But since well over half of each year's admissions was likely to remain in the asylum for some years to come, the superintendents faced the hapless task of managing an ever-greater accumulation of inmates.

In this context a danger of asylum practice was the institutionalisation of the superintendent himself. It was possible for some like Norman to put a favourable public face on this development: 'everything connected with the management of an asylum, even down to the most minute details of so-called "Administration", is a portion of the treatment of the disease, for the relief of which asylums are constructed and maintained'. This was surely no more than a rationalisation of an irretrievable situation. From another angle the matter was more critically assessed by the *Medical Press* in 1895: the asylum physician was inclined to seek in the general administration of his institution 'relief from the contemplation of hopeless masses of chronic lunacy'.[177] It was a sobering judgement on the failures of medical practice in asylums.

Notes

1. *5th Report*, p. 6, *HC* (1851), xxiv.
2. RMCB (1888-9), p. 85.
3. *51st Report*, Appendix, p. 8, *HC* (1902), xl.
4. Conolly Norman, 'A Brief Note on Beri-Beri in Asylums', *JMS*, vol. 45 (1899), pp. 503-12 and RP 1897/4876, enclosing an article in *Truth*, 11 March 1897 on the 'plague-stricken asylum'.
5. See note 3 above.
6. Cf. *Conference of Irish Asylum Committees* (Dublin, 1904), p. 56 for the evidence of Dr Mills of Ballinasloe—'it is a very common thing to have people removing their insane relatives from the asylum to work for them during the summer months'. Dr Carre of Omagh reported that this was not a practice in his district (ibid., p. 57).
7. J. Conolly, *The Construction and Government of Lunatic Asylums and Hospitals for the Insane* [1847] (Dawsons, London, 1968), pp. 140-1.
8. See above, p. 47.
9. *DJMS*, vol. 24 (1857), pp. 336-8, 342; cf. ibid., vol. 5 (1845), p. 151: an anonymous reviewer agrees with John Conolly that asylum matrons have too much power and are thus led to consider themselves independent of the physicians; ibid., vol. 27 (1859), p. 195.
10. For the rules defining the duties of asylum staff, see *11th Report*, pp. 55-8, *HC* (1862), xxiii.

11. RP 1896/9626. The honorary secretary of the union wrote to the *Daily Independent*, 15 May 1896, pointing out 'that the very head of the asylum, their medical superintendent, is a member of one of the closest trade unions that could be found in the country'. See *JMS*, vol. 43 (1896), pp. 656-8 for the meeting of doctors about the union, and *MPC*, 17 June 1896 for support for suppression of the union. Two years later an Association of Asylum Workers was formed by doctors of the Medico-Psychological Association; its annual meetings were regularly reported in the *Journal of Mental Science* and seem to indicate that no attendants were ever present. Cf. A. Walk, 'The History of Mental Nursing', *JMS*, vol. 107 (1961), p. 16.

12. *Handbook for the Attendants on the Insane*, 5th edn (Baillière, London, 1908), p. 314. The *Handbook* had first been published in 1885 by the Medico-Psychological Association. The early editions did not include this citation.

13. RP 1864/3034.

14. RP 1874/8532.

15. *JMS*, vol. 50 (1904), pp. 195-6.

16. Scull, *Museums of Madness: The Social Organization of Insanity in Nineteenth-Century England* (Allen Lane, London, 1979), p. 220 citing J.T. Arlidge, *On the State of Lunacy and the Legal Provision for the Insane* (Churchill, London, 1859). See also Scull, *Museums of Madness*, pp. 198-201 for the critique of the asylum as a machine in English psychiatry.

17. Oscar Woods, 'Our Laws and Our Staff' (address to the Psychological Section, BMA Congress, August 1887), *JMS*, vol. 33 (1887), pp. 382-4; J. Conolly, *Construction and Government of Lunatic Asylums and Hospitals*, p. 84.

18. *11th Report*, p. 23, *HC* (1862), xxiii; *13th Report*, p. 49, *HC* (1864), xxiii.

19. *32nd Report*, p. 10, *HC* (1883), xxx.

20. *15th Report*, p. 9, *HC* (1886), xxxii.

21. *Freeman's Journal*, 18 June 1873, press cutting in Larcom Papers, NLI, MS 7776.

22. *Report from the poor-law inspectors on the wages of agricultural labourers in Ireland*, pp. 1-32, *HC* (1870), xiv.

23. RP 1911/18919, a file dealing with the Asylum Officers (Employment, Pensions and Superannuation) Bill, 1911 which attempted to limit hours of work in asylums.

24. *MPC*, Irish Supplement, 25 September 1910, alleged that there was no trouble in filling vacancies but considered there was a need to guard the health of attendants by improving their conditions where necessary.

25. *Report*, p. 13, *HC* (1846), xxii.

26. RP 1848/G4508; see also RP 1847/G9207, 1849/3986, 1849/G7692, 1850/G7408 and 1851/G4439 for applications and petitions for such training.

27. *JMS*, vol. 29 (1883), pp. 459-66.

28. *MPC*, 4 December 1895.

29. See A. Walk, 'History of Mental Nursing', pp. 14-17; B. Abel-Smith, *A History of the Nursing Profession* (Heinemann, London, 1960), p. 89; for early lobbying by the MPA see *JMS*, vol 50 (1904), pp. 451-5; vol. 52 (1906), pp. 306-17, 581-4.

30. *JMS*, vol. 31 (1885), p. 149.

31. *JMS*, vol. 32 (1886), p. 122.

32. Walk, 'History of Mental Nursing', p. 12.

33. *JMS*, vol. 40 (1894), p. 491 (in his presidential address to the annual general meeting of the MPA, held that year in Dublin).

34. *Handbook for the Attendants on the Insane*, 4th edn (Medico-Psychological Association, London, 1898), p. 65.

35. Ibid., p. 67.

36. *Handbook*, 1st edn (1885), pp. 48-9 and 4th edn (1898), p. 123.

37. *8th Report*, p. 15, *HC* (1857) (II), xvii.

38. *Handbook*, 4th edn (1898), pp. 119-20.

39. *Handbook*, 5th edn (1908), p. xi. In 1923 it became the *Handbook for Mental Nurses*.

40. Ibid., pp. 314-15.

41. *JMS*, vol 40 (1894), p. 492.

42. Conolly Norman, *The Domestic Treatment of the Insane* (Dublin, 1896), p. 3.

43. RFCB (1852-87), pp. 217, 2.

44. R. Hunter and I. Macalpine, *Psychiatry for the Poor* (Dawsons, Folkestone, 1974), p. 69. The authors note that the inscription on this memorial was removed following the Mental Health Act of 1959 to 'unburden the hospital of its past'.

45. RMCB (1852-80), p. 413.

46. Erving Goffman, in *Asylums* (Penguin, Harmondsworth, 1968), analyses the characteristics of 'total institutions' and the life of the staff and inmates.

47. RFCB (1891-2), p. 665.

48. RMCB (1888-9), p. 825 (my italics); cf. RFCB (1852-87), p. 45: 'I can't elicit any delusions or hallucinations', reports the doctor.

49. RMCB (1888-9), p. 253.

50. Ibid., p. 817.

51. RFCB (1852-87), p. 17.

52. Ibid., p. 57; cf. ibid., pp. 41, 53, 221; and RMCB (1852-80), pp. 21, 241 for other comments on time.

53. RFCB (1852-87), p. 13.

54. Ibid., p. 101.

55. RMCB (1852-80), p. 9.

56. RFCB (1852-87), p. 109.

57. J. Blake, *Defects in the Moral Treatment of Insanity in Ireland...* (J.A. Churchill, London, 1862), p. 67.

58. RMCB (1852-80), p. 29.

59. See the evidence of Dr J. Robertson of the Monaghan asylum and Dr J. Lalor of the Richmond before the 1878 poor law and lunacy inquiry commission. Both made it clear that the 'incurables' were essential to the efficient and economical running of their asylums. On Robertson's calculation over one-quarter of the inmates were performing functions indispensable to the maintenance of the asylum—even if a special asylum for incurables were founded, he would need to keep most of these. *Report of the Commissioners appointed to inquire (inter alia) whether any additional and other provision is required for the better care, relief and treatment of the poor who are lunatic, idiot or imbecile in mind...* ev. 1520-9 (1837-42), *HC* (1878-9), xxxi.

60. HOS 29/1/6/2, p. 86, PRONI.

61. Cf. RMCB (1905-6), pp. 1, 37, 89 and elsewhere.

62. RFCB (1891-2), pp. 5, 153.

63. RMCB (1888-9), p. 157; RFCB (1891-2), pp. 21, 29.

64. *JMS*, vol. 33 (1887), p. 315 commenting on the poor state of the Richmond asylum. Cf. F.G. Crookshank, 'The Frequency ... of Phthisis Pulmonalis ... in Asylums...', *JMS*, vol. 45 (1899), pp. 657-83. He gives the following comparative statistics of phthisis mortality per thousand average resident population in UK public asylums, suggesting that the problem was greatest in Ireland.

	1893	1894	1895	1896	1897
England and Wales	—	14·1	15·7	13·7	14·7
Ireland	24·8	25·7	19·6	18·5	23·9
Scotland	11·0	10·5	11·2	11·6	10·4
London C.C.	12·6	9·5	12·1	8·5	9·8

See also *JMS*, vol. 48 (1902), pp. 393-434 for the report of the Tuberculosis Committee of the MPA, which includes an analysis of the statistics of Eric France (pp.

411-30), suggesting that most cases contracted tuberculosis in the asylums.

Outside the asylum, of course, tuberculosis mortality was higher in Ireland than in Britain, *Commission on Emigration and other Population Problems 1848-1954* (Dublin), para. 239 and Appendix, Table 24.

On dysentery, see *DJMS*, vol. 112 (1901), p. 429 for a report on the prevalence of dysentery in the Downpatrick asylum and measures taken to prevent it.

65. *JMS*, vol. 4 (1858), pp. 304-7.

66. *MPC*, 10 November 1847 (review of Hamilton Labatt, *An Essay ... on Restraint*, Dublin, 1847); cf. *Journal of Psychological Medicine*, vol. 2 (1849), pp. 240-62 for review of same.

67. *JMS*, vol. 55 (1909), pp. 463-4.

68. *JMS*, vol. 57 (1911), p. 627 (for a discussion of the Belfast superintendent, William Graham's paper, 'Psychotherapy in Mental Disorder').

69. *JMS*, vol. 18 (1872), p. 318.

70. Ibid., p. 317.

71. *DJMS*, vol. 120 (1905), pp. 178-9.

72. *JMS*, vol. 27 (1881), p. 333.

73. RP 1873/4734.

74. RFCB (1891-2), p. 553.

75. Ibid., p. 441.

76. Ibid., p. 497; cf. RFCB (1852-87), p. 45 and RMCB (1888-9), pp. 117-19.

77. RFCB (1891-2), p. 589.

78. RP 1879/6200.

79. RFCB (1852-87), pp. 33, 65.

80. RMCB (1905-6), p. 9.

81. RMCB (1888-9), p. 181; cf. RFCB (1891-2), p. 697.

82. RMCB (1888-9), p. 137.

83. Ibid., p. 146; cf. ibid., p. 525.

84. Ibid., p. 593.

85. RMCB (1852-80), p. 284.

86. *MPC*, 18 October, 1882.

87. *11th Report*, p. 22, *HC* (1862), xxiii.

88. *Report*, p. 23, *HC* (1846), xxii.

89. Ibid., p. 47. In 1874 the 22 district asylums had an average of 38 acres of agricultural land each. *24th Report*, p. 9, *HC* (1875), xxxiii.

90. *58th Report*, pp. xxx, xxxi, *HC* (1909), xxxii.

91. *Royal Commission*, Appendix A, p. 74, *HC* (1857-8), xxvii. Working patients received either meat with main meal or extra bread. Ibid., pp. 82-3.

92. *Report*, p. 4, *HC* (1849), xxiii.

93. *42nd Report*, p. 61, *HC* (1893-4), xlvi; *32nd Report*, pp. 20-1, *HC* (1883), xxx. See also *8th Report*, p. 74, *HC* (1857) (II), xvii. The difference between criminal and ordinary asylums in this respect is surely due to the differing financial basis of the two institutions: any gratuities to district asylum patients would have to come from the local taxpayers in the form of county rates; the criminal asylums were maintained out of consolidated revenue.

94. RMCB (1888-9), pp. 905, 773, 805.

95. RP 1857/6195.

96. RMCB (1888-9), p. 381.

97. *Royal Commission*, ev. 1508, 1666, 1887-8, *HC* (1857-8), xxvii.

98. Ibid., ev. 2999.

99. *11th Report*, p. 9, *HC* (1862), xxiii.

100. *13th Report*, p. 15, *HC* (1864), xxiii.

101. *Irish Times*, 1 August 1862 (press cutting in Larcom Papers, NLI, MS 7776).

102. *MPC*, 2 December 1857, citing report in *Belfast Newsletter*.

103. Joseph Lalor, 'On the Use of Education and Training in the Treatment of the

Insane in Public Lunatic Asylums', *SSISI*, vol. 7 (1876-9), p. 363.

104. *JMS*, vol. 21 (1875), pp. 467-74.

105. John Fox, 'On the Education of the Insane, and the School System...', *JMS*, vol. 28 (1882), pp. 16-26.

106. *Royal Commission*, ev. 2994, *HC* (1857-8), xxvii.

107. Conolly, *Construction and Government of Lunatic Asylums and Hospitals*, p.123.

108. RFCB (1891-2), pp. 301, 253; cf. RMCB (1888-9), p. 217—'his soul is lost ... all the churches are shut owing to his sins'.

109. RMCB (1888-9), pp. 909, 469.

110. See the defence of the Belfast asylum's position (probably written by Robert Stewart, the resident physician), *DJMS*, vol. 16 (1853), pp. 376-9.

111. *11th Report*, p. 6, *HC* (1862), xxiii; *15th Report*, p. 11, *HC* (1866), xxxii.

112. RP 1865/379. For their part, some chaplains accepted the criticism of preaching which over-excited its listeners or was too Calvinistic and so we get tracts such as that by W. Hyslop (of the Church Stretton Private Lunatic Asylum in England), *Cheerful Words*, being vol. II of *Sermons for the Insane* (Shrewsbury, London, 1875), see *MPC*, 10 March 1875. In the course of the Belfast dispute the rights of the medical superintendent to control the access of chaplains were in fact strengthened. The rule governing the matter in 1852 provided admission to chaplains, except where the physician declared a patient 'unfit and incapable of understanding the nature of the service, and of appreciating the effects of religion'. *Royal Commission*, p. 532, *HC* (1857-8), xxvii. But the rules of 1862 appeared to give the initiative to the doctor by requiring chaplains to administer religious instructions to those who, in the opinion of the superintendent, might be susceptible to its influence. *11th Report*, p.57, *HC* (1862), xxiii.

113. RMCB (1888-9), p. 293.

114. *Freeman's Journal*, 26 August 1864 (press cutting in Larcom Papers, NLI, MS 7776).

115. *JMS*, vol. 7 (1861), p. 29.

116. See above, pp. 155-7.

117. RMCB (1905-6), pp. 49, 145.

118. RMCB (1888-9), p. 577.

119. The asylums produced a surplus of farm and garden produce which they sold for £2,147 in 1871, £10,832 in 1911—however, they were spending considerably more than these sums in maintaining the farms (£3,098 in 1871, £27,089 in 1911).

120. *Report of the Committee ... to inquire into the Dietaries of County and Borough Gaols in Ireland, 1868, HC* (1867-8), xxxv, pp. 655-746. The report includes a survey of the diet of labourers and farmers. An estimate of Irish institutional diet in the 1890s puts expenditure on convict diet slightly ahead of that for lunatics. But the significant difference is between these diets and those in workhouses. The relative expenditure per inmate per week was given as: convict, 3s 11d; lunatic, 3s 5d; healthy workhouse inmate, 1s 5d; aged or infirm workhouse inmate, 1s 4d. *JMS*, vol. 44 (1898), pp. 106-8.

121. *Royal Commission*, Appendix, pp. 45, 81-4; *HC* (1857-8), xxvii.

122. *6th Report*, p. 9, *HC* (1852-3), xli; *18th Report*, p. 24, *HC* (1868-9), xxvii.

123. *23rd Report*, pp. 13, 38, 92, 97, *HC* (1874), xxvii.

124. *8th Report*, p. 11, *HC* (1857) (II), xvii. The inspectors' report for 1872 suggests that the wine, spirits and porter were administered only to those in hospital or under special treatment, an average per day of 330 patients. This implies nearly a pint of beer or porter per day for those receiving it, *22nd Report*, p. 26, *HC* (1873), xxx. In some English asylums beer or cider was a regular part of the diet for the inmates.

125. Cf. *JMS*, vol. 30 (1884), pp. 535-50 and *DJMS*, vol. 80 (1885), pp. 145-7 for D.H. Tuke's survey of the use of alcohol in asylums. Tuke calculated an expenditure of 14s per annum per patient in England and Wales, 8s 8d in Scotland and 4s 8d in

Ireland. This was a marked decrease since 1878 when another doctor had found the expenditure close to 30s per annum in asylums in England and Wales. See also *MPC*, 29 September, 1880.

126. D.E. Flinn, *Report on the Sanitary Circumstances and Administration of the City of Dublin with special reference to the Causes of the high Death-Rate* (Dublin, 1906). (Flinn was medical inspector for the local government board.)

127. *JMS*, vol. 32 (1886), pp. 16-22 for E.M. Courtenay's review of 'Irish Asylum Dietary'.

128. For these details of medical practice in the various asylums in 1846 see *Report*, pp. 27, 44, 30, 72, *HC* (1847), xvii.

129. *Royal Commission*, p. 16, *HC* (1857-8), xxvii.

130. *8th Report*, p. 11, *HC* (1857) (II), xvii.

131. Cf., for example, the experiments of Thomas Belgrave of Lincolnshire County Asylum on the bromides' effects on his patients, *JMS*, vol. 11 (1865), pp. 363-71; or the work of Dr Wilkie Burman with subcutaneous injections of conia (a nicotine-like drug) on himself and 25 other adults—he hoped to find 'an antidote for acute mania', (West Riding Asylum), *DJMS* (1873), pp. 425-9. The Scottish alienist, T.S. Clouston, suggested to the MPA in 1870 that empirical verification of the effect of drugs on particular classes of patients be organised. A committee of the association subsequently attempted to co-ordinate such information, *JMS*, vol. 16 (1870), pp. 24-30, and 223-9; see also *JMS*, vol. 17 (1871), pp. 278-85, for his own work on narcotics in the treatment of insanity.

132. *JMS*, vol. 23 (1877), pp. 469-70, and *Select Committee on Lunacy Law*, ev. 6867-6871, *HC* (1877), xiii.

133. *DJMS*, vol. 69 (1880), p. 244 (in a review of the article by Ringrose Atkins, the Waterford asylum superintendent).

134. *DJMS*, vol. 120 (1905), pp. 163, 165, 169-72.

135. *JMS*, vol. 51 (1908), pp. 561-75.

136. *DJMS*, vol. 77 (1884), p. 270.

137. *DJMS*, vol. 120 (1905), pp. 164, 177-8.

138. RMCB (1888-9), pp. 217, 709.

139. *JMS*, vol. 34 (1888), pp. 629-31; ibid., vol. 45 (1899), pp. 741, 799 ff.

140. For the contribution of drugs to the homogenisation of the appearance and behaviour of long-stay patients, see the comment 'Drug Effects' in R. Hunter and I. Macalpine, *Psychiatry for the Poor*, pp. 229-31.

141. As cited in Blake, *Defects in the Moral Treatment of Insanity in Ireland*, pp. 32-3; *10th Report*, p. 5, *HC* (1861), xxvii.

142. *JMS*, vol. 4 (1858), p. 539.

143. *Royal Commission*, ev. 1423, *HC* (1857-8), xxvii.

144. Ibid., ev. 8568-76.

145. *23rd Report*, p. 91, *HC* (1874), xxvii.

146. Ibid., pp. 63-4; RP 1873/12945, 1874/6284.

147. RP 1887/6865.

148. RP 1887/6828; *Hansard*, 3rd ser., vol. 314, 686.

149. *JMS*, vol 29 (1883), p. 211. In Ireland *per capita* asylum expenditure on drugs (including wines, spirit and beer) and medical appliances dropped from 11s 8d per annum in 1871 to 4s 7d per annum in 1910-11. A large proportion of this reduction would be accounted for by the great decline in the consumption of alcohol in the asylum, as has been suggested earlier in the chapter. There was a wide range of expenditure on drugs between different asylums—in 1901-2, for example, the 23 asylums spent an average 3s 6d per annum on medicines and appliances but Antrim (which had just opened) spent only 7d and Clonmel, 1s (but Clonmel had the highest level of expenditure on wines etc.) while Downpatrick spent 6s 2d and Sligo 6s 11d.

150. RFCB (1891-2), p. 749; RMCB (1888-9), p. 473.

151. RFCB (1891-2), p. 721; cf. ibid., pp. 369, 845 and RMCB (1888-9), p. 409.

152. RMCB (1888-9), p. 849.

153. RP 1873/6943.

154. RP 1889/21627; cf. RP 1899/1834 on another murder in the asylum (Ballinasloe); *MPC*, Irish Supplement 7 October 1874 (Armagh).

155. RP 1901/13212.

156. RP 1894/2664.

157. RP 1898/11666.

158. RP 1872/8861.

159. RFCB (1891-2), p. 521.

160. RMCB (1888-9), p. 817; also ibid., p. 161.

161. RP 1858/20346; 1859/9372; 1873/12237.

162. RP 1875/18618.

163. RP 1895/7596; see *MPC*, Irish Supplement, 15 April 1896 for dismissal of an attendant who cuffed a patient over the head.

164. RP 1894/6029, 1894/9718.

165. RP 1890/17632.

166. However, subsequent events vindicated Norman's concern to bring the attendant to justice. Although the government decided that the inmates' evidence was insufficient to justify prosecution, the attendant, Hayes, himself took the governors of the asylum to court for wrongful dismissal. He won his action before the Recorder but lost the appeal brought before Justice Hugh Holmes (himself the recently appointed chairman of the seven-member lunacy board of control). Holmes criticised the conduct of the Recorder in the original action (for ridiculing and discounting the evidence of asylum inmates) and observed, as Conolly Norman pointed out with some pleasure, that the evidence of the insane person can legally be accepted in a court of law liable to two limitations, viz., that the mode in which his insanity manifests itself is not such as to interfere with his evidence. RP 1890/17632; *Law Reports Ireland*, XXVIII, 107, (1890) (*Hayes* v. *Governors of the Richmond District Lunatic Asylum*).

167. RP 1891/26897; *Royal Commission*, Appendix *HC* (1857-8), xxvii; *51st Report, passim, HC* (1902), xl.

168. See Appendix, Table A; cf. Scull, *Museums of Madness*, pp. 194-8, for the same phenomenon in England.

169. Cf. *MPC*, 29 March 1882, 29 August 1888.

170. RP 1897/7092; in 1897 the Privy Council approved new regulations for the control of mechanical restraint in Irish asylums. The regulations were not welcomed without reservation by the asylum superintendents. Indeed it might be that the violence of attendants was encouraged in some way by the ambiguity of the superintendent's attitude towards the question of control and punishment. Thomas Drapes, superintendent of the Enniscorthy asylum, regretted the rigid restrictions on the use *and* temperature of the shower-bath as an instrument of punishment. See his paper 'Are Punitive Measures Justifiable?', and the discussion following it, *JMS*, vol. 45 (1899), pp. 536-49.

171. RP 1901/9759, *MPC*, 15 May 1901—the attendant was prosecuted by the government and sentenced to two months hard labour. RP 1903/10707 (Ballinasloe); *MPC*, Irish Supplement, 5 March 1902 (Cork). But see also RP 1900/15947 for the Mullingar committee which wanted an open inquiry (refused by the inspectors) into the deaths of two patients at the asylum.

172. Cf. *MPC*, Irish Supplement, 21 October 1908, 1 May 1912.

173. RP 1901/9759.

174. *Report of the Vice-Regal Commission on Poor Law Reform in Ireland*, vol. 1, paras. 159-63, *HC* (1906), li.

175. *DJMS*, vol. 118 (1904), pp. 165-6. Conolly Norman's critique of the asylum is the more worthy of notice since it came from one who was pre-eminent in his profession in Ireland. From a prominent Derry family, Norman (1853-1908) went immediately to an assistantship at Monaghan asylum on his medical graduation in 1874. After five years there he spent two years working under Dr George Savage at Bethlem Hospital in

London. His first appointment as superintendent was to Castlebar asylum from 1882 to 1885; after a further period as superintendent at Monaghan, 1885-6, he was appointed to Ireland's largest asylum, the Richmond in 1886 which he superintended till his death in 1908. He was for many years an editor of the *Journal of Mental Science* and was president of the MPA in 1894. Besides writing several papers of his own (mostly individual case studies and some on the family care system) he helped disseminate the work of German psychiatrists, particularly that of Kraepelin, among his colleagues. During his term as president in 1894 he was responsible for nominating the first woman member of the MPA, Dr Eleanora Fleury, at the time a clinical assistant at the Richmond asylum. T.P.C. Kirkpatrick biographical files, RCPI Library, Dublin; *JMS*, vol. 39 (1893), pp. 598-601; vol. 40 (1894), pp. 156-7, 691 (election of Dr Fleury defeated in 1893, accepted in 1894).

176. From the annual reports of the inspectors of lunatics, the proportion of those discharged in each year, who had been resident less than one year, to the number admitted in that year is as follows:

	1871	1881	1891	1901	1911
Male (per cent)	36·1	31·1	32·5	30·9	32·7
Female (per cent)	34·7	34·4	31·4	29·2	32·4

177. *Daily Independent*, 26 April 1892, press cutting in RP 1893/6821; *MPC*, 13 March 1895.

EPILOGUE

By 1914 the state of Irish asylums left much to be desired in the eyes of those for whom care as well as control of the lunatic was imperative. Yet political conditions in Ireland precluded the serious consideration of the status of the asylum system. At a professional level certainly, some attention had been paid to the apparent increase of insanity and the burdens this was placing on the institutions. The inspectors of lunatics, O'Farrell and Courtenay, conducted two investigations into this problem during their period of office. William Dawson, inspector from 1911, also attempted to explain the varying incidence of insanity in Ireland in a paper for the *Journal of Mental Science*, the substance of which was reproduced in an annual report.[1] Those concerned immediately with asylum management pursued the implications of the problem, chiefly from a financial point of view.[2] Nevertheless, for the reasons suggested in Chapter 2, the real political effect of this concern over increasing lunacy was to be found in the search for economies of management. A re-evaluation of the institutional order itself was left to a much later date.

In consequence to cease this study at 1914 is somewhat artificial. The features of the law and institutional arrangements that we have described remained in their essentials at least until 1945. Partition in 1921 left the asylum system in the new states largely unchanged. This was in spite of, for instance, the report of a commission of inquiry into the relief of the sick, destitute and insane poor in the Free State in 1927. This recommended the creation of auxiliary mental hospitals and observation wards and various legislative changes. Only in 1945 were the committal laws amended, removing the process from the judicial arena and placing it more firmly in the hands of the doctors, particularly of the medical superintendents. In Northern Ireland, where social policy was more subject to British influence, the end of the old 'dangerous lunatic' mode of committal came in 1932. But there too major reconstruction of the system was only achieved after the war. The tendency in both states by this time was the integration of the mental hospitals into the broader framework of the health services, thus completing a process which had begun before the Famine.

The shadow of the Victorian period was in this way thrown over the administrative and legal structures through the first half of this

century. But these have not been our only concerns. The consequences of earlier developments may have worked themselves through in more subtle ways. It is a commonplace to observe that the asylums of old have provided a poor context, a demoralising one, within which new therapies and policies might be practised. Such has been the complaint of commissions of inquiry and modern-day reformers in Ireland as elsewhere. Yet the enormous capital that is invested in institutional structures on the scale of the old district asylums makes it difficult to abandon them as the centres of social administration of the population we now call the 'mentally ill'. Boundary walls may come down, doors be opened, bars removed from windows: still the buildings remain, in some places notably isolated from the town, elsewhere surrounded by the suburbs, yet always bearing the characteristic signs of their status as centres of confinement and segregation. There is a weighty mythology about the asylum which feeds on the continuing presence of the institutions behind whose walls people are evidently powerless.

The advanced state of public provision for the insane in nineteenth-century Ireland perhaps had another perverse effect in the subsequent period. In the early 1960s the Republic of Ireland reportedly had the highest rate of psychiatric hospitalisation in the world. There are, of course, many factors involved in determining the level of such a measure. Yet as far as the provision of beds itself is concerned then Ireland was well prepared by the nineteenth century. Already in the 1850s the inspectors of lunatic asylums had been forced to defend the apparently excessive size of the new asylums: the Famine and the subsequent emigration had undermined their projections of likely demand for asylum accommodation. In spite of a continuing decline in the country's population the system continued to expand in the ensuing decades. By 1914 Ireland had a quite massive provision of asylum beds.[3] While the total population had declined by one-third since the Famine, the numbers of insane in public asylums had increased seven-fold. After the partition the population continued to decline in the 26 Counties; but there was no shortage of asylum beds for those on the margin of society. In short, the 'generosity' of nineteenth-century governments created a system which was more than adequate to deal with the casualties of twentieth-century Ireland. This apparent excess of social welfare in an earlier period may have contributed to the reluctance of Irish administrations to embark on new departures in social administration. Whatever the case, the

substantial use made of the asylum in the twentieth century was already previewed in the nineteenth.

In all regions of Ireland, in all adult age-groups and in both sexes we have seen that asylum admission rates were increasing throughout the decades to 1914. Although intended in the 1820s for the poor alone, the public asylum appeared to have an even broader social catchment by the early twentieth century. What lay reformers had viewed as 'poor asylums' were transformed by medical appropriation into 'hospitals'. The doctors saw themselves not as administering a special class of the poor, but as managers of a particular kind of illness or disease. The medical treatment was mostly an irrelevance and the medical superintendence had reverted to little more than institutional administration. In spite of this, doctors were remarkably successful in gaining a popular reputation for expertise in the diagnosis and management of insanity. By the 1890s one like Conolly Norman could report the growth of an informal consultancy service at his own asylum: hardly a week went by without some of the poor of Dublin coming to his office for advice for themselves or troubled relatives and friends.[4] Such a development signified an important transition in cultural attitudes and social practice, a growing dependence on the expertise of a professional body; in turn it encouraged the broadening of insanity's boundaries as they were defined by the doctors. Reflective doctors recognised this expansion of the boundaries, though more rarely their own role in the process. But it was a complex development, rooted also in the evolution of popular attitudes to health and illness and in the increasing role of professional medicine in everyday life. Undoubtedly the growth of popular dependence on psychiatry was encouraged by that specialty's association with a profession possessed of a burgeoning confidence in its own future. The evident failure of asylum doctors to help the majority of their charges was but a small deterrent in the face of the success of other sectors of the profession.

By 1914, therefore, the asylums were exercising an indispensable function in Irish life. In spite of their enormous financial cost, there was no likelihood of their abolition. In contrast to the detested workhouse, symbol of the humiliation of Ireland's distressed population in the nineteenth century, the asylum remained. Incorporated into the health-care services as the mental hospital, it represented the state's ongoing commitment to the management of the social outcasts, the insane.

Notes

1. See *Report on the alleged increasing prevalence of insanity in Ireland, HC* (1894), xliii; *Special Report on the alleged Increase of Insanity, HC* (1906), xxxix; W.R. Dawson, 'The Presidential Address on the Relation between the Geographical distribution of Insanity and that of Certain Social and other Conditions in Ireland', *JMS*, vol. 57 (1911), pp. 571-97.

2. Cf. *Conference of Irish Asylum Committees* (Library of the Royal College of Physicians, Dublin, 1904), and the evidence of Bishop Kelly of Ross, *Report of the Inter-Departmental Committee on Physical Deterioration*, paras. 404-7, *HC* (1904), xxxii.

3. At the beginning of 1914, Ireland had a public asylum residence rate of 490 per 100,000 population compared with England and Wales, 298, and Scotland, 283. Only a small amount of this variation can be explained by the greater provision of private asylum beds in England and Scotland.

4. *JMS*, vol. 39 (1893), pp. 308-11.

APPENDIX

TABLE A: The Expansion of Asylum Accommodation in Ireland

Asylum	Built	Number of beds					Total cost of buildings and land to 1904 in pounds
		Original	1871	1886	1896	1904	
Armagh	1824	160	162	258	408	434	117,135
Ballinasloe	1833	150	402	620	1,004	1,084	168,741
Belfast	1829	104	330	510	510	1,130	284,185
Carlow	1832	104	178	250	426	347	78,153
Castlebar	1866	260	250	355	409	419	79,273
Clonmel	1834	60	375	470	621	642	75,215
Cork	1852	500	643	709	1,173	1,286	215,550
Derry	1827	120	180	320	320	395	85,905
Downpatrick	1865	300	300	420	581	621	131,868
Ennis	1868	260	260	314	314	314	58,866
Enniscorthy	1868	300	288	316	476	457	94,055
Kilkenny	1852	152	188	290	420	420	72,335
Killarney	1852	220	220	356	556	658	82,117
Letterkenny	1866	300	300	350	510	520	96,994
Limerick	1827	150	427	500	685	673	81,827
Maryborough	1833	104	260	318	623	570	104,396
Monaghan	1869	340	340	480	807	673	123,309
Mullingar	1855	300	400	430	614	864	176,862
Omagh	1853	300	510	510	796	737	130,021
Richmond	1814	257	1,040	1,100	1,398	3,218	541,129 a
Sligo	1855	250	330	414	524	636	104,577
Waterford	1835	100	210	309	445	439	96,117

Note: a. This sum does not include the cost of the original asylum but only costs after 1830 when the Richmond became a district asylum. 1904 figures include construction of Portrane asylum within the Richmond district; Belfast 1904 includes Antrim asylum.

Source: *46th Report of the Inspectors of Lunatics*, pp. 32-3, *HC* (1897), xxxviii; *Census of Ireland, 1871, Vital Statistics*, pp. 84-5, *HC* (1873), lxxii, pt. 2; *60th Report of the Commissioners in Lunacy* (English), pp. 34-5, *HC* (1906), xxxviii.

Table B: Expenditure on Poor Relief, Lunatic Asylums and the Public Medical System, 1852-1914

Year	Poor relief[a] (in pounds)		Lunatics[b] (in pounds)		Medical[c] (in pounds)	
1852	883,267	(139)[d]	41,107	(6)	54,289	(9)
1856	576,390	(97)	77,432	(13)	90,236	(15)
1861	516,769	(90)	n.a.		104,681	(18)
1866	611,831	(111)	113,204	(20)	116,316	(21)
1871	685,668	(127)	177,395	(33)	135,005	(25)
1876	763,155	(145)	192,266	(36)	141,463	(27)
1881	965,128	(188)	206,324	(40)	157,244	(31)
1886	904,018	(184)	212,741	(43)	158,112	(32)
1891	871,424	(186)	272,616	(58)	166,330	(36)
1896	868,969	(191)	321,915	(71)	165,490	(36)
1901	976,027	(219)	427,660	(96)	173,582	(39)
1906	1,070,181	(243)	436,514	(99)	191,009	(43)
1911	1,022,125	(233)	498,939	(114)	197,068	(45)
1914	1,032,979	(238)	534,869	(123)	206,243	(48)

Notes: a. Total expenditure, on poor relief, including workhouse and outdoor relief.

b. Cost of maintenance of lunatics in district lunatic asylums.

c. Maintenance of the dispensary system (chiefly salaries of the dispensary medical officers and expenses under the vaccination acts).

d. Figures in brackets represent the rate of expenditure for each system per head of the population of Ireland in each year.

Sources: *Royal Commission on the Poor Laws and Relief of Distress*, Appendix to the tenth volume of evidence, pp. 261-2, *HC* (1910), I.

B.R. Mitchell and Phyllis Deane, *Abstract of British Historical Statistics* (Cambridge University Press, Cambridge, 1962).

Table C: Components of Asylum Expenditure, 1861-1911

Year	Salaries	Provisions	Clothing	Furniture	Fuel	Medicine	Other	Total
1861	19·5	41·6	8·9	5·2	7·0	3·6	14·2	100·0
1871	18·4	39·1	7·6	4·3	6·2	2·2	22·2	100·0
1881	21·4	41·7	9·1	4·6	6·2	2·2	14·8	100·0
1891	19·5	38·4	9·7	6·0	7·7	1·6	17·1	100·0
1901	17·8	32·5	7·5	4·1	9·3	1·0	27·8	100·0
1911	19·1	32·6	7·1	3·8	8·5	0·8	28·1	100·0

Note: 'Furniture' includes 'bedding'; 'medicine' includes wine, beer and spirits; 'other' includes building maintenance, superannuation payments, postage, etc.
Source: Annual reports of the inspectors of lunatics.

Table D: Treasury and Local Contributions towards the
Maintenance of the Insane in District Asylums, 1875-1898

Year	Treasury (in pounds)	Local Rates (in pounds)	Total (in pounds)	Treasury/total (percentage)
1875	56,948	140,469	197,417	28·8
1876	77,907	106,615	184,522	42·2
1877	80,380	130,005	210,385	38·2
1878	82,054	n.a.		
1879	84,810	103,484	188,294	45·0
1880	85,841	108,964	194,805	44·1
1881	87,250	122,679	209,929	41·6
1882	89,425	114,953	204,378	43·8
1883	92,867	122,379	215,246	43·1
1884	94,500	121,221	215,721	43·8
1885	98,698	110,008	208,706	47·3
1886	99,609	93,788	193,397	51·5
1887	101,800	104,326	206,126	49·4
1888	103,996	101,076	205,072	50·7
1889	109,118	121,158	230,276	47·4
1890	112,211	123,358	235,569	47·6
1891	111,990	146,351	258,341	43·3
1892	112,050	148,042	260,092	43·1
1893	119,721	152,838	272,559	43·9
1894	129,449	153,001	282,450	45·8
1895	126,266	164,880	291,146	43·4
1896	130,653	176,585	307,238	42·5
1897	137,511	183,815	321,326	43·0
1898	143,653	216,742	360,395	40·0

Source: *64th Annual Report of the Inspectors of Lunatics*, p. xxix, *HC*
(1914-16), xxvi. Figures are available from 1899 onwards in this source,
but are not continuous with this series as they include provision for loan
repayments for capital works.

Table E: Dangerous Lunatic Committals as Percentage of all Admissions

Asylum	1868		1871		1891		1911	
	Male	Female	Male	Female	Male	Female	Male	Female
Armagh	88·6	89·7	76·5	80·5	77·7	68·2	34·5	10·0
Ballinasloe	80·0	69·0	90·5	74·4	84·2	75·3	66·6	56·8
Belfast	73·3	44·4	50·7	49·2	51·8	27·8	91·7	94·2
Carlow	35·8	38·0	56·6	45·0	53·5	50·0	56·6	46·6
Castlebar	53·5	65·3	53·4	53·8	78·6	87·8	95·3	90·1
Clonmel	60·0	50·0	60·9	33·3	67·3	52·9	66·6	60·3
Cork	37·5	25·5	67·2	56·8	83·5	85·9	61·1	53·2
Derry	25·8	31·5	68·7	32·8	74·4	58·0	60·0	49·0
Down	—	—	42·0	35·5	56·3	36·4	64·2	36·5
Ennis	28·9	0·0	43·4	52·0	76·0	60·0	98·2	94·7
Enniscorthy	14·0	40·0	43·4	32·4	50·0	46·8	54·0	43·5
Kilkenny	71·4	54·5	60·0	6·6	89·4	83·8	55·5	62·5
Killarney	74·3	67·8	68·0	48·4	84·4	81·3	90·0	95·1
Letterkenny	66·6	34·1	77·0	64·1	87·6	87·5	90·9	91·8
Limerick	26·1	11·1	28·3	40·8	62·7	65·8	79·3	75·7
Maryborough	38·2	28·1	41·0	18·4	62·7	43·1	52·9	45·2
Monaghan	—	—	65·8	47·8	96·2	98·1	93·4	97·5
Mullingar	73·7	27·7	72·8	43·1	83·7	87·0	91·3	80·8
Omagh	25·3	35·7	35·1	24·6	87·2	89·7	86·8	86·1
Richmond	48·9	40·0	63·3	46·8	78·7	73·8	66·6	39·5
Sligo	0·0	0·0	71·0	44·1	87·8	87·8	86·6	87·3
Waterford	50·0	70·2	25·7	17·9	41·4	16·2	75·0	46·1

Note: Down and Monaghan asylums were not open in 1868 and formed part of Armagh district. The separate district of Antrim in 1901 and 1911 is included with Belfast.
Source: Annual reports of the inspectors of lunatics.

Appendix

Table F: Asylum Admissions and Residence Rates, 1844-1914 and Workhouse Admission Rates, 1858-1914

Year	Asylum admissions[a]	Workhouse admissions[b]	Asylum residence[c]
1844	7·9		31·1
1845	9·0		30·7
1846	9·1		31·4
1847	13·0		32·3
1848	11·8		33·6
1849	12·2		35·2
1850	13·0		37·5
1851	14·5		41·7
1852	18·1		45·2
1853	19·2		49·2
1854	18·0		54·2
1855	25·4		60·4
1856	20·9		64·5
1857	21·7		66·9
1858	22·1	22·9	69·4
1859	22·3	19·6	71·2
1860	21·6	22·8	73·6
1861	n.a.	28·5	75·8
1862	20·2	38·7	77·9
1863	21·2	42·0	81·7
1864	18·2	37·6	83·8
1865	18·5	36·0	86·4
1866	25·8	33·4	91·7
1867	23·3	38·5	94·3
1868	38·7	44·1	106·4
1869	42·8	34·0	115·9
1870	35·9	33·8	122·8
1871	34·5	33·5	129·5
1872	33·2	35·3	132·8
1873	34·7	38·8	137·8
1874	33·2	39·6	143·1
1875	33·6	32·0	146·6
1876	35·7	26·6	152·9
1877	36·3	29·8	154·8
1878	36·6	38·9	159·1
1879	37·1	49·1	161·2
1880	36·9	61·0	166·5
1881	39·7	61·0	174·4
1882	41·8	55·8	181·7
1883	43·4	51·2	189·9
1884	44·4	50·9	194·7
1885	45·3	55·6	199·8
1886	43·6	64·4	205·4
1887	46·1	70·6	216·1
1888	45·6	73·2	225·4
1889	48·9	68·6	235·0
1890	51·9	61·7	243·4
1891	50·2	57·8	250·7
1892	52·1	59·5	261·8

Year	Asylum admissions	Workhouse admissions	Asylum residence
1893	53·3	61·7	269·8
1894	53·3	62·6	278·2
1895	53·9	60·5	292·3
1896	56·4	64·7	309·1
1897	56·3	68·5	322·2
1898	59·2	73·9	338·4
1899	63·4	n.a.	353·3
1900	62·0	71·0	367·0
1901	63·4	62·1	379·5
1902	71·5	71·8	396·3
1903	70·7	75·4	409·5
1904	70·7	74·6	422·3
1905	67·4	83·3	433·2
1906	62·8	94·1	438·9
1907	62·5	92·8	444·6
1908	69·9	100·4	456·9
1909	64·7	100·2	462·0
1910	64·8	96·9	469·8
1911	67·2	93·1	476·6
1912	62·6	96·5	484·3
1913	61·4	86·5	490·4
1914	64·5	85·1	496·7

Notes: a. Admissions per 100,000 mid-year population: 1844-62, all admissions; 1863-1914, first admissions.
b. Admissions per 100,000 mid-year population. Figures prior to 1858 not available in a continuous series.
c. Numbers resident at end of year in district asylums, per 100,000 mid-year population.
Sources: Annual reports of inspectors of lunatics, 1844-1914.
Annual reports of local government board, Ireland, 1872, 1899-1914.
B.R. Mitchell and Phyllis Deane, *Abstract of British Historical Statistics* (Cambridge University Press, Cambridge, 1962).

Table G: District Lunatic Asylums—Discharge, Re-admission and Death Rates, 1851-1911

	Discharges[a]		Re-admissions[b]		Deaths[c]	
	Male	Female	Male	Female	Male	Female
1851	17·1	18·2	n.a.	n.a.	7·6	6·4
1861	13·7	16·2	19·6	16·8	6·9	6·0
1871	14·4	15·6	17·4	16·6	7·0	7·0
1881	12·8	13·5	19·3	21·9	6·8	7·6
1891	12·7	12·4	23·1	21·2	6·1	6·8
1901	9·4	8·8	22·0	19·2	6·3	6·5
1911	7·7	7·4	21·9	21·0	5·9	6·2

Notes: a. Discharges as a percentage of total population treated during year (resident at beginning of year plus admissions).
b. Re-admissions as a percentage of all admissions.
c. Deaths as a percentage of total population treated during the year.
All rates calculated on a three-year average (that is 1850, 1851, 1852, etc.) except 1861 (33 months to 31 December 1861).
Source: Annual reports of inspectors of lunatics.

Table H: District Lunatic Asylums—Age Structure of Admissions, Deaths, and Discharges, 1889-1893

Age	Male (percentage)			Female (percentage)		
	Admissions	Discharges	Deaths	Admissions	Discharges	Deaths
0-10	0·1	0·0	0·0	0·0	0·0	0·0
10-15	0·7	0·0	0·4	0·7	1·0	0·2
15-20	6·8	6·7	1·9	7·2	9·3	2·3
20-25	14·7	14·9	6·5	12·8	14·1	5·7
25-30	15·1	14·6	8·7	13·2	14·6	9·8
30-35	12·5	13·3	10·8	12·4	11·6	10·0
35-40	10·4	11·2	8·6	10·8	11·6	9·8
40-45	8·8	9·5	10·7	10·6	9·7	9·8
45-50	7·7	7·7	10·3	9·3	9·5	10·4
50-55	6·9	7·4	9·1	8·0	7·1	11·0
55-60	5·0	5·1	8·9	4·8	4·1	7·5
60-65	4·5	3·9	7·3	4·2	2·9	7·9
65-70	2·0	1·4	5·9	2·0	1·7	5·7
70-	2·7	1·0	9·8	2·3	0·8	8·7
Unknown	2·1	2·1	1·0	1·7	1·3	1·2

Source: Annual reports of the inspectors of lunatics.

A NOTE ON SOURCES

The principal source for study of asylum policy and administration is the *Chief Secretary's Office Registered Papers* (State Paper Office, Dublin). The contemporary indexes to the papers include a register of the correspondence of the lunatic asylums office. As will be evident from its use in this book, the correspondence included material relating to policy, planning, finance and administration of the asylum system from 1845 to 1921, as well as inquiries into the history of individuals committed to the institutions. Although necessarily selective, these inquiries frequently contain details of nineteenth-century practice unavailable in the routine records maintained in asylums.

These records of central administration must be supplemented by the parliamentary reports of the inspectors. The annual reports, printed in the *House of Commons Papers*, contain the aggregate statistics of the institutions as well as occasional reports on the status of individual institutions and the various asylums. Studies of particular hospitals would require use of the official *Minute Books* of the board of governors, later the committee of management. These survive in some hospitals in the Republic and, for some Ulster institutions, at the Public Record Office in Belfast.

Most of the prominent figures in asylum administration were only second-ranking parliamentarians and officials and private papers throwing light on their activities tend to be rare, not only in Ireland. An exception in the Irish case is the collection of material relating to lunatic asylums in two volumes of the *Larcom Papers* (National Library of Ireland); unfortunately, Larcom was Under-Secretary during a period of only secondary importance in the history of asylums in the nineteenth century, so this source is of interest chiefly for its unveiling of Dublin Castle at work.

Apart from an occasional appearance in the official papers in their role as asylum administrators and managers of the insane, the preoccupations of the doctors are to be found principally in the medical journals. Three are of interest in the Irish context. The *Journal of Mental Science* (founded in 1855) was the professional organ of the asylum superintendents, organised from 1841 in a body known later as the Medico-Psychological Association. Irish doctors

were active in the association from the 1850s; the journal contains articles by some of them as well as, from 1873, reports of meetings of the rather low-key Irish branch of the association. As the principal British voice of the emerging specialty of psychiatry the journal is indispensable for understanding the ideological context of asylum treatment in this period.

Two Irish journals supplement this specialist journal. The *Dublin Journal of Medical Science* (founded in 1846) had a broad compass but occasionally brought within its range the concerns of asylum work. From the 1870s this journal included a review of contemporary research in psychological medicine and physiology. The *Medical Press and Circular* (originally the *Dublin Medical Press*, founded in 1839) contained frequent news items on Irish asylums and from the 1870s there was an Irish supplement (the *Irish Poor Law and Lunacy Intelligence*) which provides some information about lunacy committals by dispensary medical officers.

For information about life in the asylum, about the practice and preconceptions of 'psychological medicine' in its everyday aspect, we are of course heavily dependent on the asylum records. These also are the way into the experience of the insane themselves, their histories before committal and their lives within the asylum. The state of preservation of these records, where they have survived, has not been good in the Republic; in Northern Ireland, where they have been under the control of the Public Record office, the records are much more complete. Three types of records provide significant information about the insane and their experience, and might form the basis of more detailed local study than has been possible for this general survey. *Admission warrants* were required for all patients committed under the Dangerous Lunatics Acts, *house forms* for all others. Where these are in near complete preservation (for example, for Omagh asylum, Public Record Office, Belfast) they can provide a picture of typical patterns of committal and of any changes over time, for a particular district. *Admission registers* (available, for example, for Omagh and Belfast, PRO, Belfast and Sligo, St Columba's Hospital, Sligo) contain basic biographical data for all those admitted to the hospital and would be equally useful in the context of a local study. *Case-books*, while also containing biographical data, are more important for examining both medical attitudes and behaviour, and reactions of patients to their experience of the asylum environment. The extent to which such information is accessible through the case-books varies from place to place: the Richmond case-books, used

extensively in Chapter 5, are particularly rich in recording the behaviour and even language of the inmates as compared to the Belfast books which are more routine and cursory in their reporting. It goes without saying that these sources, recording as they do the lives of people who would not otherwise have left traces of their history, should be indispensable for social history. Although necessarily a selected population, the asylum inmates shared many characteristics and experiences of their peers; information about them in asylum records will therefore touch areas of interest beyond the boundaries of this study: family life, structure and conflict, the experience of the aged, the contexts of drinking and drunkenness, the disappointments and anxieties of the rural and urban poor in nineteenth-century Ireland.

INDEX